COMPLETE GUIDE TO
EYECARE, EYEGLASSES & CONTACT LENSES

Psalms 103: 3

Renewmy youth like the Eagles

REVISED
FOURTH EDITION

Thank you God

Undipling Thoughts

COMPLETE GUIDE TO
EYECARE, EYEGLASSES & CONTACT LENSES

Walter J. Zinn
and
Herbert Solomon, O.D.s, F.A.A.O.s

REVISED
FOURTH EDITION

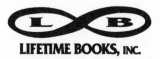

LIFETIME BOOKS, INC.
2131 Hollywood Blvd., Suite 305
Hollywood, FL 33020

Library of Congress Cataloging-in-Publication Data

Copyright 1996
Zinn, Walter J.
    The complete guide to eyecare, eyeglasses, and contact lenses /
Walter J. Zinn, Herbert Solomon. -- [4th ed.]
        p.   cm.
    Includes index.
    ISBN 0-8119-0821-6   : $14.95
    1. Eye—Care and hygiene—Popular works. 2. Eye—Diseases.
3. Ophthalmic lenses. 4. Ophthalmology—Popular works.
I. Solomon, Herbert. II. Title.
RE51.Z56   1996
716.7—dc20

Printed in Canada

Photographs on pages 148 and 175 courtesy of Bernell Corporation, South Bend, Indiana.

Contents

Foreword

The idea for this book was first spawned in the lobby of a dinner theatre where Neil Simon's "Gingerbread Lady" was playing. Herb Solomon's wife, Phoebe, an accomplished actress, was appearing in the play. Walt Zinn, a professional photographer in his teenage years, was casually invited to take publicity photos of the players. We (including Zinn's wife Barbara) attended the weekend performances during the run of the show. Many topics were discussed between acts, and somehow, the conversation turned to writing a book on vision care.

We were both aware that the great majority of people are relatively uninformed on this subject. Because of that ignorance, we were disturbed and exasperated—many people were receiving less than adequate care without being any the wiser. It was and still is our hope that a comprehensive, easy-to-understand book will encourage people to seek out better professional services.

By the end of the show's run, we had an outline, effervescent enthusiasm, a budding camaraderie, and the painful realization that writing for a lay audience is no easy task. Concepts that we could easily express in professional jargon, became nearly as difficult to put into simple a language as balancing the federal budget.

We often argued like the "Odd Couple." It was necessary to perform a marriage of the minds combining our experience, background and writing styles into one palatable approach. Walt Zinn has the lighter writing touch; Herb Solomon is a stickler for the minutest detail. We spent about twenty-five hours a week writing, discussing, rewriting, rethinking and rewriting. Because of our mini-debates, respect for each other's talents and knowledge increased.

Those of you who dabble in astrology would contend that we enjoyed the provocative mental stimulation because we are both Geminis. Perhaps so. But whatever the reason, we certainly did enjoy it. We hope the reader, too, will find it provocative, informative and gain a fuller appreciation of the many facets of optometric vision care.

—1977—

Seven years after the above was written, it is pleasant to report that we are still colleagues and good friends. There have been a few sad occasions, but blissfully many joyous ones— graduations, marriages, births...lots of births! The Solomons have been happily and tumultuously involved with seven grand children which easily eclipses the Zinn's one granddaughter.

Our fascination with science of vision and our interest in optometry have not diminished. There are so many projects we have planned (research, lectures, writing), that it should keep us busy for years. That thought is delightfully invigorating.

—1986—

Eight more years have passed and the third edition of the book with many revisions and additions has been completed. You might think it gets easier each time, but not really. The same attention to detail, researching the latest information and putting it into easy-to-understand language, is still a painstaking process. Despite the time expended in the writing which could have been used for well-deserved leisure time, it never entered our minds to do otherwise. We enjoyed doing it seventeen years ago and still enjoy the process.

On the birth front, the Solomons are up to twelve grand kids. The Zinns have narrowed the ratio with two grand daughters. In 1986 it was seven to one; now it's six to one. The Zinns hope that trend continues.

—1995—

It is very gratifying that the third edition of our book sold out in just one year. During that year we have gotten older, but merely to keep up with the general aging population; we'll leave "and wiser" to the discretion of the reader.

When our editor telephoned to request additional material for this edition, we plunged into the writing with our usual zeal. It's an enthusiasm sustained by the conviction that people want to understand their eye and vision problems, which means presenting it in a language devoid of jargon, and explanations devoid of gibberish. That has always been our goal and we continue to operate on that basis.

Doesn't it seem like the pace of everything is picking up? The computer revolution has certainly seen to that. It has made possible new diagnostic and treatment options not dreamed of when we wrote our original book. Despite the ongoing changes in the health care field which create additional pressures on the individual doctor, we both continue to practice optometry in our private office settings. That's the way we like it.

—1996—

Walter J. Zinn, O.D.,F.A.A.O.
Herbert Solomon, O.D.,F.A.A.O.
Morton Grove & Glencoe, Illinois

I

Your Visual World

1

What's Your Vision All About?

The odds are 99 to 1 that you need eye care now or will need it in the future. Your life style, your occupation and even your life depend on good vision. You get more information about the world through your eyes than all your other senses combined. Yet, vital as it is, you tend to take your vision for granted because most of the action takes place behind the scenes. What do you really know about your eyes and how you "see?" Why do you have two eyes instead of one or three? How do you see colors? Why must the two eyes work together? What can a cataract do to your sight? Are your "sunglasses" doing you more harm than good? How do you know if your toddler or child has good vision?

You probably have less information about your vision than you do about vitamins, angioplasty, or diets. If you are the average person, you worry more about your teeth than about your eyes, probably because toothaches can be painful and teeth can fall out. Well, poor vision doesn't ordinarily hurt, although it may be disguised as a headache, fatigue or avoidance of near tasks (the child who "hates" to read); and eyes rarely fall out.

Most parents will anxiously drag a (protesting) child to the dentist twice a year to check for cavities, poor bite, protruding teeth, etc. That's fine. But these same parents are not consciously aware that neglecting a child's vision may lead to graver consequences than an impacted tooth—namely, poor schoolwork, limited job choices later in life, or even blindness.

In a long-overdue and gratifying action by the legislature of the State of Illinois, comprehensive, professional eye exams are now required for students entering designated grades. This is a far cry from the previous double standard which mandated professional dental exams, but trusted the results of eye "screenings" administered by lay persons. Other states should copy this laudatory legislation.

Consider this quote: "The demands upon our eyes in our days have greatly increased over those made by our ancestors ... The demands upon school children's eyes have been excessively increased in the last years."

Does this sound appropriate? It was written in 1894, a century ago, by Dr. St. John Roosa, Professor of Diseases of the Eye and Ear, New York Medical School and Hospital. It was written before electric lighting made reading for many hours into the night a general practice; before television and movies; before automobiles were driven at high speeds (or even at all); before fifteen years of schooling was common (and many more years for advanced degrees); before computer screens populated offices and homes; before the era of technological miniaturization and millimicron tolerances.

All these activities are dependent on good vision, and as far as the natural evolutionary development of the visual system is concerned, most of them are highly artificial and "Johnny-come-lately's".

Is extreme sharpness of sight necessary to milk a cow? Do you need binocular vision to stomp on grapes to make wine? Does a crossed or a "lazy" eye prevent you from planting corn, feeding livestock, shoveling manure?

Undoubtedly, modern civilization puts demands on our eyes and visual system for which they were not naturally designed. We treat many patients who have symptoms of discomfort, headaches, doubling of vision, etc. which are directly attributable to the patient's occupation or life style. There is not too much we can do about the way our modern technological society is run. (While we may yearn to return to simpler, bygone days, few of us would be willing to give up all the conveniences, benefits and comforts we enjoy.) Modern civilization is here and we are stuck with it for better or for worse. But, we must carefully watch the abuse our eyes are taking in the process!

Small deficiencies in clarity, differences in the way the two eyes see, poor focusing ability, or lack of good stereoscopic vision may not matter much in a slow agrarian society. They will, however, play havoc with an individual's effort to manage with the contemporary world of school, occupation, sports, etc.

What you are about to read in the following chapters is a comprehensive discourse of the marvel we call vision, the many problems which can beset you eyes and vision, how they can be alleviated, or made more tolerable. The information is geared to cover not only all the questions lingering in your mind, but to help you make new and fresh discoveries.

2

Do You See What You're Looking At?

Your flippant answer to this question would be: "of course." A couple of examples and a few minutes of thought might change your mind. Look at the illus tration below. What do you see?

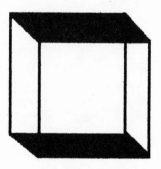

Do you see what you are looking at?

This is the familiar Necker cube. If you look steadily at it, the figure will flip-flop; the front surface becomes the back surface and vice versa. The changes are spontaneous and out of your conscious control. Try as you will, you cannot keep the box in one orientation. (It's called a Necker cube for the simple reason that the Swiss naturalist by the name of L. A. Necker first described it in 1832.)

You might protest that this is an unfair example because it's an illusion. Indeed it is—a visual illusion as contrasted to an optical illusion. (The difference is explained in Chapter 6.) Far from being an isolated and unique sensory event, the Necker cube perfectly dramatizes that all vision is an illusion created in the brain. The visual system must always and continuously make rapid determinations as to object size, distance, motion, shape, color, etc.

Notice, please, that we use the term "vision" and not "sight". Sight is the input from the eyes; vision is the resulting perception you experience in the brain. In fact, this chapter should be titled "Do You Vision What You Are Looking At?" but it sounds clumsy.

Let's consider the difference between sight and vision. The well-known Rorschach "ink-blot" test used by psychologists makes an excellent example. Everybody sees the shape and design of the figure, but it represents various things to different people. This is the crux of the point—vision is interpretation of what the eyes see.

However, even without full interpretation you can store an artist's depiction in the brain and quickly recognize it the next time. For instance, there is a famous Picasso sculpture standing in front of Chicago's City Hall. There are many guesses, but nobody truly knows what it's supposed to be. Yet, it's instantly recognizable to anyone who has ever seen it. In this case, the visual system interprets it as "that Picasso sculpture".

Going a step further, do you really know what you look like? Most people don't. Sure, you see yourself in the mirror, but that's not the way others see you. (We're using the word "see" but you should be thinking "vision".) The image in the mirror is reversed which accounts for the unfamiliar view of yourself in home videos where the image is not reversed.

The difference goes deeper than that, however. "Beauty is in the eyes of the beholder" is an almost correct adage. If you substitute the word "brain" for "eye" it might not sound as romantic, but it would be scientifically more accurate. Assuming normal sight, the image the eyes receive is about the same for most people. What the brain does to interpret that image could make a big difference between individuals. Experience, culture, and emotions all enter into what you visualize. The visual system of a four-year old child living in Los Angeles instantly interprets that moving configuration as an automobile; the visual system of a four-year old living in an isolated Brazilian jungle village would not.

We can't be certain if everyone visualizes colors the same way. Even discounting those people with known color vision problems, does red look the same to everybody? Color is very much a part of our experience and culture. It's unlikely that you would be comfortable eating a green steak.

You now begin to appreciate that seeing and vision are not the same and are subject to many variables. In fact, except for basic innate functions, meaningful vision is a learned process which takes place in the brain from stimuli generated in the eyes. If we factor in nearsightedness, farsightedness, astigmatism, poor eye coordination, disease, color deficiencies, etc., we may indeed ask: Do you see (vision) what you are looking at?

3

The Eye

Without a doubt, the eye is our most important sense organ, accounting for about 80% of our awareness of the environment. Moreover, it is the only sense organ without any distance limitation. Touch and taste are obviously contact senses; smell and hearing have a limited range and lack precise localization. Yet, you can look up at the night sky, locate and see a galaxy so very far away that its light may have taken thousands of years to travel through the universe. Without any apparent fuss, your eye can also localize and see objects a few inches from your face with great detail.

Your eye can see in very bright sunshine and in almost total darkness, spanning a huge range of illuminating on the order of a million to one. It can see a rainbow of colors and, with its partner eye, can see objects in solid depth. It can detect the slight stirring of a bird among the uncountable leaves on a giant oak and can track moving objects with uncanny precision.

To be accurate about it, the eye doesn't achieve all these remarkable exploits by itself. Ultimately, they are accomplished by the eye's commander, advisor and controller—the brain. Before discussing that segment of the story, let's have a closer look at the structure and functions of the various parts of the eye.

THE EYEBALL is roughly a sphere about an inch in diameter brimming with many specialized structures and tissues. The round shape is ideal for easy rotation within the bony orbit. In cross-section it looks like this:

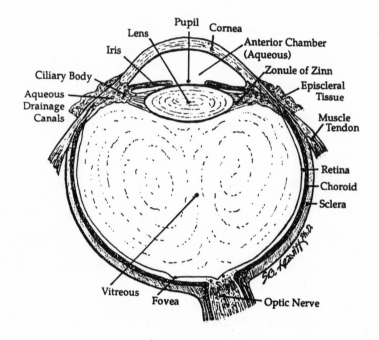

THE CORNEA is a transparent tissue covering the very front of the eye much as a watch crystal covers the dial. Besides being transparent, the cornea is devoid of blood vessels and is highly selective in its sensitivity. (The last point is important for contact lens wear.)

THE IRIS is a circular curtain composed mostly of tiny, radial muscles which contract and relax to shape the size of the pupil. It's the colored part of the eye. A person's eye color depends on the number of pigment cells in the iris; light blue has the least, and dark brown has the most.

THE PUPIL is a hole in the center of the iris which looks black because the inside of the eye is dark. (The "red-eye" effect in flash photography is simply the pupil as seen with light reflected off the retina.) Its size varies with the amount of light entering the eye, your age, focusing tone, etc.

THE LENS is a transparent, elastic, semi-soft material about ½ the diameter of a dime which can change shape to focus on objects at different distances from the eye. It is suspended in place by threadlike fibers called the Zonule of Zinn (alas, not named after one of the authors). The fibers are connected to the ciliary muscle. To focus at a close object, the ciliary muscle contracts loosening the fibers' tension on the lens and allowing it to bulge. This increases the optical power of the system.

As the lens ages it loses some of its elasticity and cannot bulge as much. This is known as presbyopia (aging eyes) and is the reason people, beginning in their 40s, tend to need reading glasses.

THE VITREOUS HUMOUR is a clear, jelly-like substance which fills the rear two-thirds portion of the eye. The small space between the cornea and lens is filled with a clear, watery AQUEOUS HUMOR.

THE RETINA is the paper-thin tissue lining the inside back of the eyeball. It's composed of specialized light-sensitive cells, several layers of a variety of typical brain-type cells and a network of arteries and veins across the surface. A comprehensive study of the retina is outside the scope of this book. We'll deal with those aspects which will help you to understand vision and vision problems.

In cross section, the retina is a formidable complex system of interconnected nerve cells. Looking at the illustration you realize that the retina seems to be inside out, counter to what you'd expect intuitively. Photons of light have to travel through all the layers before they can impact the receptor cells. Some of the light is even blocked by the blood vessels and never reaches the sensory layer. One reason may be that the light sensitive cells have to abut the dark pigment layer which prevents light scatter and performs nutritional functions.

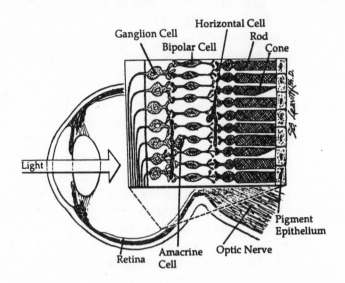

A diagramatic view of a tiny section of the retina showing its many layers and complexity of nerve cells.

If you recall a bit of basic biology, the light receptor cells are the rods and cones, so named because of their shape. The rods are much more numerous and very responsive in low illumination. The cones can distinguish finer detail and see colors but at the penalty of needing more light. (In the dark all colors look the same because only rods are stimulated.)

The cones are packed closely together in the center of the retinal expanse in a small region called the macula, only 1/10th of an inch across. At the hub of the macula is a tiny depression, the fovea, which is the locus of sharpest sight. It's an almost infinitesimal 1/40th of an inch across. When you "look" at something, you turn your eyes so that the light rays are focused precisely on the fovea. Keep this point in mind when we discuss crossed and "lazy" eyes.

In all, there are over 130 million light sensitive cells in the retina of each eye; about 125 million rods and about 6½ million cones. Most of the cones are concentrated in the macula; the foveal cramming is 147,000 per square millimeter which is one of the reasons this spot has the keenest sight. (For perspective, compare this to a good laser printer at 5,500 dots per square millimeter.) The fovea enjoys two other advantages: 1. There is very little overlying retinal layers, or blood vessels to obstruct the light rays; 2. Cones have a more direct wiring circuit to the brain.

The foveal sight is quite sharp, but since it's so tiny it's very limited in scope of view. Only a small area of a scene can be focused onto the fovea at each glance. The illustration below demonstrates it.

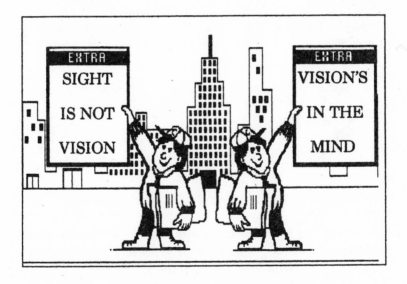

Your field (expanse) of vision is quite large, but the span of distinct sight is very small. To read the words you must shift your eyes to each one in turn. Example: When looking at the word SIGHT you're aware of words to the right, but to identify them, your eyes have to "jump" there.

Why so many cells in the retina? Millions of bits of information must be gleaned from a typical scene in a fraction of a second. Some population of cells are organized to distinguish only very distinct patterns. For instance, some will only signal a black vertical line on a light background; others a black horizontal line; still others for oblique angles. There are some groups which signal borders, but only borders in a particular orientation. Other arrays of cells respond to motion, but only one explicit direction of motion. While all this is going on, there have to be cells which respond to colors, to forms. You now begin to grasp the complexity of the retina where all these things have to happen in a split second.

Approximately 1 million nerve fibers carrying electrical impulses generated by the retinal cells (estimated at about 1 billion bits per second) leave the eye via the optic nerve. At its attachment at the back of the eye this 1/4th of an inch diameter area is devoid of visual cells and is, therefore, blind. That's the normal blind spot of the eye. The illustration below will prove it to you.

With the left eye closed, stare at the X at about 14 inches and slowly bring the page closer. At a certain distance the face will disappear as its image falls on the blind spot.

The blood supply for the inner layers of the retina enters at the optic nerve. The vessels divide and branch out to overlay the retinal surface. It's the only place in the body where blood vessels can be seen (by the doctor looking into the eye) in their natural condition.

SIX EXTRA-OCULAR MUSCLES attach to the outside of the eye to govern movement. Think of them as divided into three pairs with each set working in opposition to each other. For instance, contraction of the medial rectus and relaxation of the lateral rectus will point the eye inward. The eye movements are so habitual that you're hardly aware of them. The teamwork among the muscles must be precise and accurate. They must also match and coordinate with the movements of the other eye. Since there is no connection between the muscles of the two eyes, the coordination is done by nerve signals from the brain.

THE EYELIDS protect the delicate cornea from foreign particles and, by blinking regularly, keep a layer of tears on the cornea. The tear film is produced by glands within the lids. A bone dry cornea would quickly loose its transparency.

4

Why Two Eyes?

Since most of the organs of the body are paired, you might have taken your two eyes for granted. If you stop to think about possible reasons, you might decide that with two eyes you can get a wider field of view to the sides. True enough. But to have a really terrific field of view, wouldn't you design the system to have one eye mounted on a finger-like stalk atop your head to see all around? Wouldn't it be nice to have the ability to see behind your back? The way it is now, there has to be a elaborate neck joint complex so that you can turn your head to get a reasonable near-360 degree panorama. Yet, nature evolved into our present set-up. Why?

Actually, by itself, a very wide field of view is not all that beneficial. While it's good for noticing movement and general shapes, it's very poor for seeing details. (Try threading a needle out of the "corner" of your eye.) Seeing movement is adequate for a frog since it merely triggers a reflex action to catch a fly, but for us it's important to know what caused that movement. Is it a charging rhinoceros or only the shadow of a bird? To make this vital decision we must see it in detail. Why can't we see in detail over the entire field of view? Very simply, the limited size of the brain.

As you will recall from the previous chapter, the retina's area of detailed sight is the macula which is about 1/20th of an inch in diameter. The flood of nerve signals from this tiny area alone keeps a large part of the brain occupied with interpreting the visual meaning. (The visual cortex allocates about 35 times as much space to the fovea as the rest of the retina.) If the entire retina had the sight property of the macula, the eye would have to be much bigger and the brain logarithmically larger (room-size). It's doubtful if you could even "attend" to so much information.

Our vision is actually an adroit compromise. To the sides we have a reasonable field of view without much detail; at the macula we have a very limited view with marvelous detail.

It would be possible, though, to have this arrangement with just one eye bulging out of the center of the forehead. That's impractical because the eye would be very susceptible to injury. So the eye is placed within a bony vault for maximum protection. If you put your mind to it, you could come up with several alternate placements for the eyes—fore and aft, for instance. But there is a very distinctive advantage to frontally placed eyes with overlapping fields of view—depth perception.

Before you say, "Is that all?," remember that nature thinks so much of stereoscopic vision that a very elaborate system is involved to produce it. The retina is divided almost exactly down the middle with the nerve fibers from the outer half of each eye connecting to the same side of the brain; the nerve fibers from the nasal side cross over and connect on the opposite sides of the brain. This seems like a curious arrangement, but it's not the crossing that's curious (your left hand is controlled by the right side of the brain). The nerve fibers which don't cross are part of the secret of depth perception.

Because the eyes are about two and one-half inches apart, each retina receives a slightly different image. You can easily prove this if you hold your finger 8 inches in front of your nose and alternately close each eye. The position of the finger will seem to shift back and forth. Within the brain there are special cells which match the offset images from the two eyes to yield the sense of solid depth.

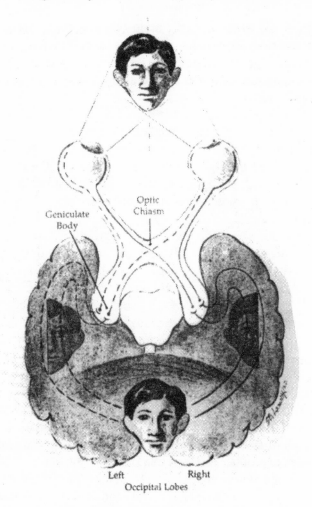

Geniculate
Body

Optic
Chiasm

Left   Right
Occipital Lobes

A diagramatic view, looking down at a cross-section of the eyes and brain, showing how the nerve fibers cross over.

The nerve fibers from the two right halves of the retina end up on the right side of the brain; the left halves end up on the left side.

The two half-images are "welded" into one by the brain. We do not normally see the half images as shown in the drawing.

However, in certain cases of brain injury or disease, it is possible that only half the field of view will be seen.

There are other ways to see depth which can be achieved with only one eye: perspective, size, surface texture, shadows, etc. which are all employed to depict a sense of three-dimension in pictures. But it is simply not quite the same as true stereopsis.

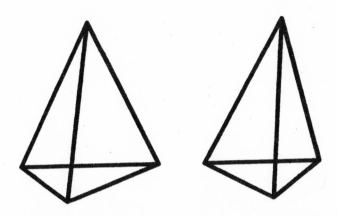

Stereopsis. *By crossing or uncorssing your eyes you can fuse these two images into a single solid pyramid with depth. To cross your eyes, make believe you're staring at a spot in front of the page. To uncross your eyes, look at a spot between the two images and make believe you're looking far away. When crossing the eyes, the pyramid will appear smaller and the point of the base will be further away.*

Is stereopsis all that important for survival? It's difficult to reconstruct exactly how much advantage it conferred on our ancestors. Certainly, grasping and picking up objects is much simpler with 3-D. Whatever the reason, nature labored long and hard to perfect it, so let's enjoy it.

As with any system, the more complicated, the more potential there is for errors. To appreciate the full value of depth perception (and for it to develop), very precise and intricate alignment of the eyes is essential. Horizontally, the alignment must be within a few degrees of arc; vertically, much less. If the six muscles controlling each eye cannot point the two eyes at the same spot within this narrow range, the stereoscopic effect will be diminished or lost. The very narrow range of vertical alignment explains why people who develop a condition wherein one eye sights slightly higher than the other, will often see double.

5

"I See," Said the Brain

If you've followed along so far, you understand that we have two eyes sending billions of electrical bits through the optic nerve to the visual cortex of the brain. This is where the ultimate action takes place. Somehow (and researchers are slowly beginning to unravel the mystery), the brain interprets these signals into a stable, colorful, three-dimensional world out there.

You realize, of course, that the brain does not actually "see" the tiny, two-dimensional, upside-down, distorted and constantly shifting image on the retina. No light reaches the brain at all; it only receives patterns of nerve impulses from which meaning must be rendered. We usually do this so effortlessly (apparently) that the very complicated nature of the process is difficult to appreciate and decipher.

For purposes of this book, we will highlight some of the more intriguing aspects.

The fact that the image on the retina is upside-down seems to puzzle some people as to why we don't see that way. But remember, the brain is not looking at the retina. It constructs the visual world so that down is where your feet are normally planted, up is towards the sky within a general frame of reference. If you stand on your head, the scene looks "unusual" but the chair is not standing on the ceiling.

21

A   B

C

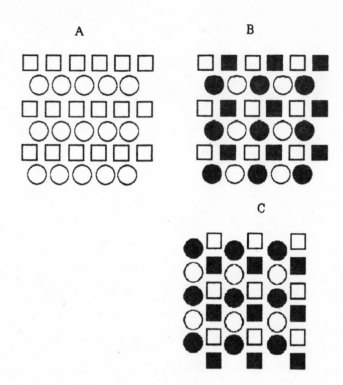

PATTERN SETS AND CAMOUFLAGE

In (A) the boxes and circles are instantly organized by the visual system into horizontal patterns.

In (B) the pattern has been disrupted by merely filling in every other box and circle. That's the principle of camouflage.

(C) is B rotated 90 degrees which makes an organized pattern re-appear.

A more difficult idea to reconcile is that the eyes are in constant motion, yet we see the world as a stable entity. The eyes continuously jump about, quickly shifting from one location to another in fractions-of-a-second, ballistic hops called saccades. How can the brain get any meaning from a perpetually changing image on the retina? Surprisingly, the changes are necessary for vision. The cells in the retina and visual system respond best to changes with a rich outpouring of signals -- changes in brightness, color, texture, orientation, etc. Without these changes, there would be no vision!

Try this experiment. Stare at any object and make a mighty effort to keep your eyes perfectly still. It's very difficult to do, but if you can manage it you'll notice that parts of the scene begin to fade away. Chances are you'll make an involuntary, slight eye movement because the brain will not easily tolerate loss of vision.

Scanning is vital for recognition. When you see something for the first time, the brain will try to match it section by section with stored memory images. Curves and angles are very important as major clues. Think back a moment. The first time you looked at a new automobile model, you had to look carefully and at length so that the brain could absorb and store the new configurations. The eyes made rapid saccades, lingering longest on the most modified parts. Once this information is stored in the brain, you can recognize the auto in almost a single glance even if it's a different color.

Each eye sends a separate image to the brain, but you usually see only one object. Want to see more? Hold your thumb up at arm's length and sight across it at a distance object with both eyes open. You not only see two thumbs, one from each eye, but also the single image of the distant object. What's going on? The answer is tied up with the essence of depth perception. There are special brain cells which have the ability to combine similar objects located within a limited, prescribed range of the two eyes into one percept. When this is achieved, the individual images are squelched. In the above experiment, your thumb images are outside the operating range of these cells.

So far we've been discussing looking at still life objects. Suppose we now complicate matters by having the object move. The images flit around on the retina just as they do when the eyes move. How does the brain know the difference? Assume you're riding on a train. How does the brain decide if the telephone poles are moving or if you're moving? In all such instances the brain must also factor inputs from other sources such as the neck muscles, legs, etc., then make a reasonable guess based on past experience. Most of the time the decision is correct, but sometimes the brain is fooled into a visual illusion. (You're on a train in a station next to another train. The other starts to move and you're convinced yours is moving.)

Want to make the world move? You can by introducing a type of eye movement the brain never encounters. Place your finger on the outside lower lid and gently push the eyeball while the other eye is closed. Now the world does move because the brain has no experience at integrating the push of the finger. We wonder how many such pushes it would take for the brain to learn to veto the sensation of movement.

It makes simple geometric sense that you can tell the size of an object by the size of the image on the retina. Indeed, there is very little relationship. A person's face twelve inches away may project onto the entire retina while that same face across the room will create an image on only five percent of the retina. Yet, you don't see the former as the face of a giant. The brain applies what is known as size constancy. If you know the size of an object the brain will "see" it that way regardless of the image size on the retina. Size constancy is very necessary for maintaining order in our visual world.

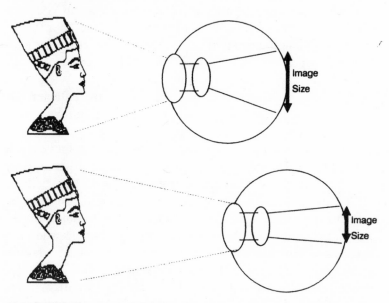

SIZE CONSTANCY. *Though the images on the retina change size depending on the distance of the object, the brain makes the compensatory adjustment so that we see it in its "true" size.*

If you want to prove to yourself that retinal image size has little bearing on what you see, try this experiment. With one eye closed stare are a light bulb for about ten seconds in a darkened room. Turn the bulb off and blink several times to create an afterimage. Look at a piece of paper 12 inches away. The afterimage will be a certain size. Now look at the wall across the room and the afterimage will be much larger even though the retinal image never changed.

Another way to maintain order is shape constancy. (See illustration below.)

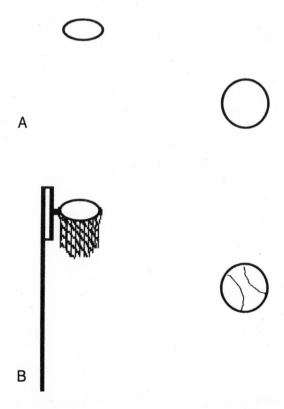

In (A) it looks quite obvious that the circle cannot fit through the ellipse. In (B) the circle becomes a tossed basketball and the ellipse is the hoop. With this persective, the circle will easily fit through the ellipse.

If you know the shape of something, you see it that way regardless of the retinal image. Have you ever taken a photograph pointing upward at a skyscraper? Undoubtedly you were disappointed by the distorted shape -- the top almost comes to a point and the windows get smaller and smaller. When you look at the skyscraper directly, the image on your retina approximates the same distortion as on the photo, yet you see it as a normal building, not coming to a point with tiny windows near the top. That's shape constancy because from experience you know what a building looks like.

The remarkable brain doesn't need complete images to get vision. It fills in the blanks from memory and experience. Just a few lines on a piece of paper will elicit visual meaning. Look at the drawing. Do you have any trouble "seeing" (after we tell you) that it's a bird's-eye view of a straw-hatted man riding a bicycle?

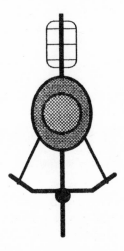

Do you see a straw-hatted bicycle rider?

Still more remarkable, the brain doesn't even need a drawing. Just the word "elephant" conjures up a visual memory. However, if you don't know what a duck-billed platypus is, there is no visualization.

This gives you some flavor (albeit, minor) of the complicated workings that go on in the visual system before the brain can say: "I see!"

6

Visual Illusions

et's get one point cleared up right away—a visual
illusion is not the same as an optical illusion. The
latter is caused by an outside device, usually optical
(hence the name): a lens, prism or a mirror. For instance, a telescope produces an illusion of enlargement; a
mirror (or reflection in water) may produce an illusion of an
upside-down scene. A hologram is an illusion which produces
a life-like image in space.

But, a visual illusion is created within the visual system, not
externally. It is the result of the brain's normal struggle to make
sense out of the information it received from the eyes, information which is frequently scanty, unreliable and may be in
conflict with information arriving from the other senses.

You are aware from the previous chapter that the visual cortex not only extracts meaning from, but places its own interpretation on the signals coming from the eyes. Often there are
several possible ways of interpreting the total flow of information into the brain. What it comes down to is that the brain
must make a "best bet" decision of what you are looking at.

For example: Suppose that on a clear, summer night you are
gazing up at the stars. Suddenly, the star pattern image on your
retina begins to rotate like a giant pinwheel. The brain has only
a fraction of a second to decide whether the heavens are spin-

ning, the world is spinning or you are spinning. The "best bet" is that you are whirling.

We can turn this setting into a visual illusion by actually rotating the heavens. It can be done, and routinely is, in a planetarium where the projected star patterns can be made to whirl. When this happens, the brain "best bets" that you're in a spin and you'll grasp the arms of the chair to keep from falling off. Even though your other senses may tell you that you're sitting still, the powerful visual sensation wins out.

Most common visual illusion, some of which are pictured here, are artificially created by a drawing which is itself an artificial creation. Pictures and drawings make use of visual clues to induce the brain into thinking that you're looking at a real object with real depth.

By injecting perspective in drawings, such as converging lines and different sized objects, the illusion of a real scene is evoked. By altering the normal perspectives, false illusions are created. So-called "impossible" pictures depend on such creations plus the fact that you can only scrutinize a small portion of the picture at a time.

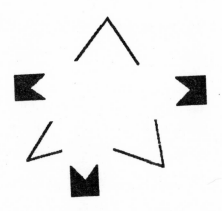

VISUAL ILLUSION. *The apparent white "Overlay" figure is not really there.*

Some illusions are merely indicative of the way the visual system organizes the inputs for easier interpretation. The tendency is to group objects into sets or patterns.

As you might imagine, motion can induce illusions. When you drive along at night, the moon seems to follow you. Why? Even though you know intellectually that the moon is a quarter of a million miles away, the retinal image makes it appear as a large disk only a few miles away. While other objects of the same apparent size (a building, stand of trees) are soon by-passed, the moon is still in the same place. This could only be possible if, indeed, the moon were traveling along with you. Because the brain makes this assumption, that's exactly what you "see". There is another moon illusion which has not yet been explained satisfactorily -- the fact that the moon at the horizon looks much bigger than the moon high up in the sky.

The size of an object also influences your judgment of its speed. The moon seems to move much slower than the 65 miles per hour that you're driving. If you've ever watched airplanes land, you are quite convinced that the giant 747s come in much slower than a small airliner. Their real speeds are almost the same.

The more detail in a scene, the easier it is for the visual system to correctly identify the physical objects. Conversely, the fewer the clues the brain has to work with and the more assumptions it has to make, the more likely an illusion. That's why most real-life illusions occur at night under dim light conditions, particularly when there is motion involved. Most UFOs are reported at night.

The occasional illusions we experience are the price we have to pay for a very flexible visual perception system. Retinal images are used mainly to trigger previously stored images in the brain. This is much more efficient than having to laboriously study each object every time it appears. A charging grizzly bear doesn't wait for a leisurely inspection by the eyes. Most often the "best bet" is a winner; on rare chance the wrong stored depiction is presented -- presto, an illusion.

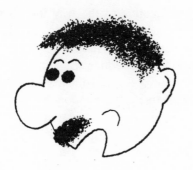

VISUAL ILLUSION. *A normal caricature until you examine it closely and realize that both eyes are on the same side of the nose.*

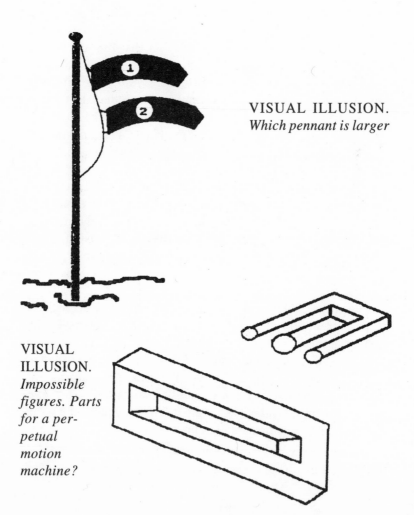

VISUAL ILLUSION. *Which pennant is larger*

VISUAL ILLUSION. *Impossible figures. Parts for a perpetual motion machine?*

7

Color Vision

To be absolutely truthful about it, there is really no such thing as physical color. There are only various wavelengths of light which give rise to a sensation of color in our visual system. You might, if you were given to puns, call it a pigment of the imagination. Yet, we do see in colors like fish, birds and other animals which have this remarkable gift.

There are a few theories as to how color vision works. None are completely satisfying because the exact mechanism is unknown. But, it is well established that there are three separate cone receptors in the retina for each of the primary colors—red, green, and blue. By mixtures of these three in sundry combinations we see all the colors. This is known as normal trichromatic color vision.

For example, a yellow flower will stimulate both the green and red receptors to signal the brain in a code which it recognizes as "yellow". Purple is a mixture of red and blue, and so on, with all possible hues.

The wavelengths of light to which our eyes respond are a tiny fraction of the entire electromagnetic spectrum. These wavelengths are measured in nanometers (billionth of a meter). The blue cones have their peak sensitivity at 440 nanometers; green at 535; red at 570. The overlap and proximity of sensitivity of the green and red cones helps explains why most people with color vision problems have difficulty with red /green tones.

The mixing of colored lights to produce another pure color is a very unique property of the visual system. Musical notes cannot be mixed to obtain a pure third note. But colored lights mix completely and there is no way to see its components. Yellow is the most striking example. It's made up of green and red, but you see no trace of either.

(A note to artists: Mixing colors of light is not the same as mixing paints. Mixing red, green and blue light produces white light; mixing red, green and blue paint produces black.)

If you've learned anything at all from the previous chapters you know that nothing is simple in the visual system. The three receptors in the retina do begin the process but, as usual, the brain takes over. We've mentioned size constancy and shape constancy to which we can now add color constancy. Somehow, we see colors correctly despite the difference in amount and quality of light. The brain factors in the surrounding colors and borders to maintain consistency.

People who have difficulty recognizing colors are commonly said to be color blind. The term is very inaccurate. Only very few individuals are so totally color blind that the world appears to them like a black and white movie. This very rare condition is usually in company with other vision defects and very poor sight.

Generally, color blindness is really a color deficiency which makes particular colors or certain pastels hard to recognize. About 7% of men have some form of color deficiency; only 0.5% of women are affected. It is a genetic defect, always affects both eyes, and doesn't change appreciably during a lifetime. There is no known cure.

The commonest type of color deficiency is the eye which uses all three primary colors but in the wrong proportions. Such people need brighter colors for recognition. Pastels are quite allusive. During times of fatigue or stress, even bright colors may be misjudged. If you have one of these persons around the house, he is always setting the TV with too much red or green.

Another type of deficiency is the person who uses only two of the three primary colors. Such an individual will be "red blind" or "green blind". "Blue blind" is extremely rare. The red blind individual doesn't see red and oranges as the normal person does. Those hues look dark grey or even black. An orange or red traffic sign could look about the same. All purples look like blue because the red part of the mix is not detected. To the green blind person, red, orange and green all look similar and even have the same brightness.

It's possible to acquire color deficiencies as the result of disease or aging. For instance, barbiturates used as sedatives may cause changes in yellow-green vision; excessive use of caffeine will alter the sensitivity to all colors. The aging eye will see things more yellowish when the lens loses its clarity.

Because color is used extensively in the classroom, color vision should be checked at an early age. Pity the green blind boy who is told by the teacher that all the nouns are on the pastel green cards and all the verbs on the pretty orange cards. He's lost before he begins.

Another reason for early detection is to help in choosing a career. Occupations such as chemists, painters, interior decorators, engineers, etc. rely heavily on good color sense. The individual should be aware of any potential difficulties.

II

How Your Eyes Should Work and What Can Go Wrong

8

Normal Focusing and Eye Movements

The long and elaborate chain of events which ultimately results in conscious vision begins in the eye. Nothing can happen until an image is formed on the retina. The brain gets the most reliable information when the image is sharp and clear, with crisp borders and angles. The clearness of the image is referred to as visual acuity and that's where the familiar 20/20 comes in.

What does that fraction really mean? It's based on a formula of visual angle (20/20 = 5 minutes of arc) devised by a fellow by the name of Snellen in the last century. The acuity chart uses specific size letters (or numbers) at 20 feet. The top number of the fraction is the distance at which you can see the letters; the bottom number is the distance at which you should be able to see the letters. For instance, 20/40 means that you see at 20 feet what you should be able to see at 40 feet. 20/100 means you see at 20 feet what you should be able to see at 100 feet.

Some doctors use the metric equivalent of 6/6 meters. In either case the chart's distance is not an arbitrary figure, but the least distance at which the eye's near-focusing mechanism is virtually at rest.

For a few minutes let's forget that the eye is a living organ and only consider it as an optical system to focus the outside world onto the retina. The word "refraction" is indispensable in this discussion, so let's define it.

Light rays/waves normally travel in straight lines. Refraction means that the light rays are deflected when they pass from one transparent medium into another of different density. The simplest way to understand this is to place a spoon into a glass of water and look at it from the side. The spoon seems to be broken at the surface of the water and at the rim of the glass. It's because there are three different transparent mediums, air, glass and water, and the light rays are deflected—refracted— when they cross the borders.

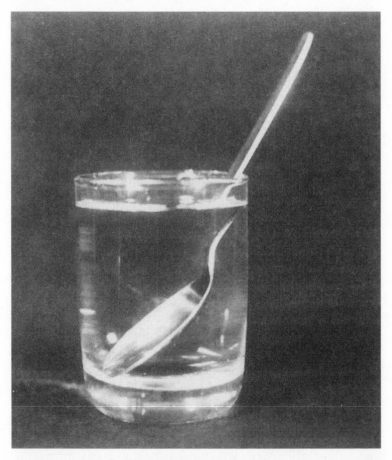

The spoon appears broken at the edge of the glass and at the water line because both glass and water bend light rays more than air.

The eye has several transparent mediums of differing densities through which the light rays pass to reach the retina. The greatest amount of refraction takes place at the surface of the curved cornea which is much denser than air. (If you've ever opened your eyes under water you've noticed that vision is blurry. The water, being denser than air, creates an altered refractive balance.)

The lens within the eye is another major refractive body. But, while the cornea has a fixed contour, the lens is able to modify the amount of refraction by actually changing its shape. It is, in effect, a variable focusing system to bring light rays from an object to a sharp focus regardless of its distance from the eye.

Here's how it works. When you look at something at least 20 feet away, the lens maintains its minimum curvature and least light-bending power. When you look at something closer, the lens will become more bi-curved and thicken to increase its refractive power and bring the light rays to a sharp focus. This lens focusing is called accommodation and is triggered by a blurry image on the retina. (See Figures A and B on page 40.)

A very important point is that both eyes will accommodate the same amount. The two eyes cannot work independently.

If the overall refractive power of the eye exactly matches the length of the eyeball, a perfectly focused image is formed (ignoring, for the moment, the normal distortions). Being a living organ, there are many possible variations in the eye's refractive parts. A minor discrepancy in the radius of the cornea by as little as 1/10th of a millimeter or in the length of the eyeball by 1/3rd of a millimeter can throw the image out of focus.

Assuming that a sharp image is focused on the retina, it must also be focused on a very tiny, specific spot. The eye must keep the image centered on the fovea for best sight. This is no simple task when you realize that the eye is constantly moving and what you're looking at may be moving.

The brain is engaged endlessly in a hunt and find game to keep the eyes positioned correctly. A steady stream of nerve signals is sent to the external muscles of the eyeballs. Matching signals are sent to both eyes so that they work in unison. Normally they cannot work independently. (With practice you

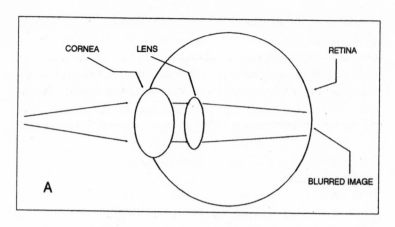

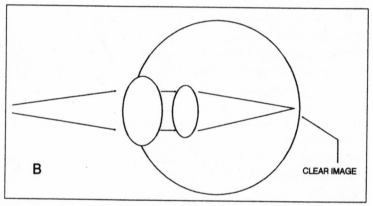

ACCOMMODATION. *For reading at near or to see things clearly at close range, the lens of the eye has to increase its curvature (bulge) to focus the light rays onto the retina. If it did not as in (A) the rays would focus "behind" the retina and the image would be blurry. In (B) the lens has adjusted the focus to place the light rays exactly on the retina for a clear, sharp image.*

With increasing age, the lens loses its pliability and can no longer focus near objects. For most people this occurs in the 40s; reading glasses or bifocals are needed.

can learn to rub your tummy and pat your head; no amount of practice will enable you to move one eye up and down while the other is moving back and forth.)

But, hold on, things get even more complicated. There are two basically different eye movements: (1) Both eyes move in the same direction, i.e., to the right or down; (2) The eyes converge, turn inward, to keep an object centered on the foveas. All these movements occur simultaneously with almost unlimited combinations. As you read this, your eyes are sweeping right and left, probably looking downward, while they are also converged.

It's quite easy to demonstrate convergence if there is another person handy. Hold a pencil about 20 inches in front of his or her nose and slowly advance the pencil towards the nose. If the person keeps watching the pencil you will see the eyes converge, turn inward. A person with good convergence should be able to follow the pencil to within about 3 inches before one or both eyes swing outward.

Looking at near objects or reading requires both accommodation of the lens and convergence of the eyes. Evolution of our visual system has linked these two functions together. A given amount of accommodation pulls a given amount of convergence with it, and vice versa. It's economical for the nervous system, but since there are variances in living organs, it leaves the system wide open to all sorts of problems which will be discussed in later chapters.

9

Common Sight Disorders and Corrections

There are four common refractive problems of the eye. A refractive problem exists when the image is not properly focused on the retina. This occurs in hyperopia (farsightedness), myopia (nearsightedness), astigmatism, and presbyopia (aging eyes). Emmetropia describes an eye without a refractive problem.

HYPEROPIA: The hyperopic or farsighted eye is essentially too short (from corneal surface to retina) for the refractive power of the eye. Hence, the light rays from any distant object would theoretically come to a focus behind the retina which, of course, can't happen because the retina is in the way. If you've ever focused a slide projected picture onto a screen, and then moved the screen closer, the picture is out of focus. That's the case with the hyperopic eye—the retina (screen) is too close.

For the brain, the blurred image on the retina is similar to the blurred image when a normal eye looks at something close up. So, the brain signals the lens of the eye to accommodate (increase power) to bring the focus forward onto the retina. While this automatic system is designed for seeing up close, the hyperopic eye uses it for distance seeing. It works rather well as long as the amount of farsightedness is not excessive and the lens remains flexible. Hyperopic people can generally see quite clearly at distance. (Actually, with small amounts of hyperopia, the eye's distance seeing could be excellent because the mild focusing reduces some aberrations.)

There is one major drawback, however. Since a portion of the near-focusing capacity is used for distance seeing, less is available for close seeing. If the hyperopic individual is required to do a lot of reading or detailed close work, the extra strain may induce fatigue and headaches. Even without a lot of reading, as the person get older and the flexibility of the lens is lessened, distance sight will also become blurry.

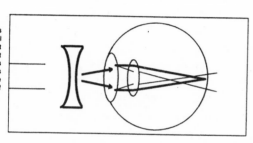

The nearsighted eye is corrected by an optical lens which is thin at the center and thick at the edges. This diverges the light rays to compensate for the excess convergence of the eye.

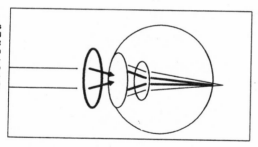

The farsighted eye is corrected by an optical lens which is thin at the edges and thick in the center. This converges the light rays to compensate for the inadequate convergence of the eye.

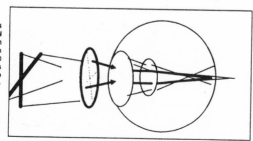

The astigmatic eye is corrected by an optical lens which is thick in one meridian and thin in the meridian 90 degrees away. This compensates for the divergent and convergent effect of the eye.

If the eye is very farsighted, even in young people who have large measures of focusing ability, distance sight will be affected. In this case or if symptoms are present, glasses or contact lenses will be prescribed. Many times it may be adequate to use glasses only for close seeing.

MYOPIA: The myopic eye is too long for its refractive power. The light rays come to a focus in front of the retina, then spread out to form a blurry image. Contrary to the hyperopic eye, there is no way for the nearsighted eye to clear the image. (Lens focusing would only increase the blur.) Myopic people can see things clearly if they are reasonably close and reading is usually not a problem. Squinting helps a bit in seeing far away because the narrowed opening sharpens the image. Glasses or contact lenses will be prescribed to enable the person to see distant objects.

There are many theories for the development of myopia. We know that nearsightedness generally shows up in a child of primary-grade age and continues to increase during the growing years. (See Chapter 32.)

ASTIGMATISM: This is a common disorder, but very difficult to explain. If any of the refractive surfaces of the eye are not symmetrical, parts of the image are clear, parts blurry. Looking at a tiny spot of light, the astigmatic eye would see a blurry streak. The culprit is usually the surface of the cornea (although it could be the lens and even possibly, the retina). Instead of being perfectly round like the surface of a balloon, the cornea is slightly oval as when the balloon is squeezed. Astigmatism causes distortions in the image. You can get the idea by looking into an oval teaspoon and noting the distorted reflection caused by the out-of-round shape.

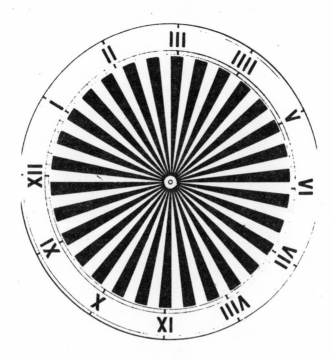

Look at this clock wheel with one eye covered. If some of the spokes appear blacker than the others, you have astigmatism.

The same kind of distorted image is formed on the retina. But, while it may be blurry and indistinct, the person is not aware of the distortion because the brain "straightens" the perception. Therefore, an intriguing thing happens. When the astigmatism is corrected with glasses, the person will see clearly, but often complains of objects being tilted and out of shape for a few days until the brain recalculates "straight." Uncorrected astigmatism can cause headaches and eye strain. Frequently it's an additional complication to hyperopia and myopia.

PRESBYOPIA: "Aging eyes" catches up with most people in their 40s. The first symptoms include difficulty in reading small print, threading a needle, having to hold a newspaper at arm's length, etc.

If you look at the graph, it's evident that as the lens of the eye ages, its focusing ability decreases. For most people, the critical age is 45. Why? To read at 16 inches requires 2½ diopters of focusing which is just about what the 45-year-old has available. Using all of it quickly tires the system. Holding the

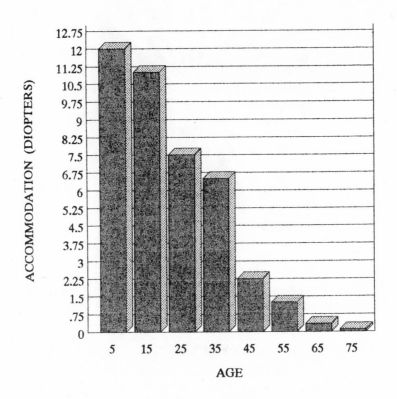

The relationship between age and focusing ability. There is a steady decline in accommodation as you get older which eventually demands your use of reading glasses or bifocals.

print at 20 inches reduces the demand to 2 diopters which can be dealt with for a short reading session. Holding the print still further, say 26 inches, can get you by for a longer time since only about 1½ diopters are needed.

Farsighted people are affected at an earlier age because they use up some of the focusing for far seeing. A succinct description of presbyopia would be: The brain is willing but the lens is not fully responsive and your arms are too short. That is, the brain continues to send signals to the lens to accommodate, but the lens cannot comply as it did when it was younger. Glasses will be prescribed to compensate for the reduced ability of the lens to focus. These can be in the form of reading glasses or bifocals.

TWO EYES: While it is possible for both eyes to have the same refractive condition, it seldom happens, although they're usually similar. If they differ greatly and the difference is not corrected early enough, a host of other problems including amblyopia and/or crossed eyes may result.

III

The Eye Examination

10

How To Choose A Family Optometrist

Perhaps we should first ask: "Do you need a family optometrist?" If you're the type of person who has a family dentist and a family physician, your general eye care should be provided by a family optometrist. It ought to be a primary care optometrist, not an ophthalmologist. The primary care optometrist is, by training and experience, qualified to diagnose, manage and treat conditions and diseases of the human eye and visual system as regulated by the laws in your state; also to recognize and diagnose related systemic disorders. The ophthalmologist is a secondary or tertiary provider, basically a surgeon concerned with diseases and injuries of the eye. If there is an indicated need of those essential services the optometrist will advise you. It's the same idea as your dentist telling you when you need a peridontist, or your physicians referring you to an orthopedic surgeon. The optometrist is the general vision care specialist and is the one to consult when you have a vision problem. Sooner or later you will need eye care, so you might as well be prepared.

Choosing a family optometrist is about as easy or difficult as finding any other professional person to suit your needs. In the last few decades this problem has been exacerbated because we live in such a mobile society. With every move of a substantial distance, you have to go through the process all over again. It's almost traumatic. (If you currently have good professionals in any field, ask them to recommend people in your new location.) The phenomenal proliferation of health care plans such as Health Maintenance Organizations (HMO), Preferred Provider Organizations (PPO), and others which at first blush seem to resolve the issue, really do not, as we'll discuss later. (The National Health Care scheme is a total unknown at this time.)

The problem is really two-pronged: 1. Finding a very competent person; 2. Finding someone with whom you can feel comfortable. We can offer some help and tips to avoid the most obvious mistakes and make your search a little easier.

As a starting point, you could ask friends and neighbors for a recommendation. Ask someone whose opinion you respect. There is no guarantee that you'll like the optometrist, but it's certainly worth investigating.

A more objective starting point would be to contact the American Academy of Optometry—(301) 718-6500 and request a list of members in your state. To become a Fellow of the Academy (F.A.A.O.), the optometrist must demonstrate firm clinical skills and knowledge. This does not imply that without being an F.A.A.O. the practitioner cannot be qualified, but with those initials, competence is almost assured.

Another starting point might be to contact the state optometric association. Each state has its own association which is affiliated with the American Optometric Association. It will be listed by the name of your state, i.e., Arizona Optometric Association, New Jersey Optometric Association, etc. They will generally provide you with several names in your geographic area.

If the above two suggestions are not feasible, you can, as a last resort, look in the yellow pages under "optometrist." Be forewarned, however, that finding an optometrist this way is like picking a winner at the race track by closing your eyes and sticking a pin into a name. You just might come out lucky, but the odds are not good.

Every optometric office receives phone calls from people who "let their fingers do the walking." Can you guess what the most common question is? "How much are..." followed by the words "contact lenses", or "bifocals", or "colored contact lenses", etc. No reputable professional can possibly answer that question without knowing anything about your condition, what type of bifocals or contacts are suitable, whether you could use them, and so on. Anyone who quotes a price in advance is probably just enticing you into the office. Does that mean you shouldn't ask any questions? It only means you should ask substantive questions. Here are some suggestions:

Q. How long has the doctor been in practice?

- If you have a choice, pick someone with more experience.

Q. How long has the doctor been in that practice/office?

- The optometrist might have graduated 25 years ago, but has shifted around every few years. A warning flag.

Q. How much is the general examination fee?

- The answer should be a range depending on specific tests you might need.

Q. Does the doctor regularly attend continuing education classes?

- Self evident.

Q. Is the doctor a member of the American Academy of Optometry?

- A good sign of competency.

Q. Does the doctor lecture and/or write on optometric topics?

- Obviously, not everyone can be a lecturer or needs to be a lecturer, but you can decide.

Q. Will the doctor examine an 18-month old toddler?

* That's a bit of a trick question, especially if you don't have an 18-month old. However, the answer is very revealing because it indicates the doctor's level of expertise and willingness to spend time with you.

To elaborate on that last question, it's possible that the doctor just isn't interested in examining infants and young children. That's O.K. But, the answer you get should not demean the importance of an infant's exam, and should indicate a readiness to refer to someone who does. You can also make up your own question regarding any specific problem you have. Don't be surprised if a series of such questions confounds the receptionist at the other end of the phone line.

To improve your odds of getting sensible responses, by all means AVOID box or display ads. The larger the ad, the less likely it's someone suitable for you. Look for a simple name listing; if it includes Fellow, American Academy of Optometry, so much the better. Steer clear of "cutsie"-named places such as Bright & Shining Eyes, Sore Eyes Fixed, Upscale Contacts, etc. (Just as you should steer clear of Happy Smile Dental, Teeth Are Us, or Pretty Baby Pediatrics.)

Specifically, you should look for an optometrist in private practice whose NAME is his/her reputation, who will treat you as an individual and is interested in your problem. The office should be pleasant, the staff friendly and the equipment must be modern. A very useful rule of thumb is to estimate the allocation of office space: make certain more space is devoted to testing than to frame displays. It's a good indication where the main interest of the optometrist is centered.

When you read Chapter 12, The Vision Examination; What It Must Include, you'll be in a better position to judge the testing procedures itself. If there's anything you don't understand, ask. The optometrist should discuss your problem and how to solve it. If the answers are short or incommunicative, get yourself another doctor.

Considerable advertising is done by some optometrists, by optical departments of retail stores, and especially by national optical chains. These chain operations spend tens of millions of dollars via television, radio, newspapers and direct mail to lure you into their stores. The sales pitch will vary: "$10 off"; "free frame with purchase of lenses" and the asterisk tells you in tiny print what the conditions are; "Trust us, we care." You can be certain of one thing—they care about the profit, and very little else.

(The silliest and most insulting idea to the consumer is "glasses in about an hour" as if that's the only thing that matters—the quality of the examination and thoughtful diagnosis is irrelevant. Is there no time allocated for the examination? Notice, it never states: "Allow 45 minutes to an hour for the exam." If we project their frivolous logic further, would it be four times better if you could get glasses in about 15 minutes?)

The competence of the optometrists in these establishments is open to question; frankly, it's a crap-shoot. They are commonly under the direction of a nonprofessional person. These lay merchants have found that they can make a substantial profit by marketing glasses and contact lenses just as they might merchandise shoes or washing machines. The optometrist merely functions as a necessary salesperson, nothing more.

Even if the optometrist is competent, it is unlikely that he/she can devote the time necessary for a complete examination of about 45 minutes, because time equals money. The corporate employer is not concerned with your eyes and vision (despite what is cleverly claimed in the ads), except with how much earnings your vision problem can generate. Since advertising is very costly, a high volume of traffic is necessary to sustain its price tag plus producing a profit. If you are foolish enough to blunder into such a place, you will be hustled in and out of the examination room in a hurry. The examination likely will be cursory and the diagnosis could be incomplete or faulty. A poor diagnosis can sometimes overlook a serious or life threatening health hazard. The number of people patronizing these stores is a sorry testimonial to the willingness of the general public to accept mediocre services (of all kinds).

Every professional field, sad to say, has individuals who are only interested in the dollar. The oath taken upon graduation or licensing, to put the interest of the patient foremost, is pretty much consigned to the dust bin. You have one advantage in the case of these optometrists and optical chains—it's really easy to tell who they are because they advertise themselves!

A fairly recent innovation is the "referral service" which will "find you a suitable doctor" by calling a telephone number. Essentially there are two types: 1) operated by a hospital or 2) by a commercial enterprise. Obviously, the hospital-run service will provide you with only the names of the doctors on the staff. The commercial enterprise will provide you with the names of doctors who have paid to have their names listed. Think of it as yellow pages advertisements in a different format. It's a poor option.

Advertising has its place and uses, but not in professional activity. Some years ago the Illinois Supreme Court ruled on a ban on optometric advertising by saying "...the legislature is not dealing with traders in commodities but with the vital interest of public health and the treatment of bodily ills. The public is concerned not only with the maintenance of standards which will insure competency of the individual practitioner, but protection against those who would prey upon a public peculiarly susceptible to imposition through alluring promises of physical relief. In addition, the community is concerned in providing safeguards not only against deception, but against practices which tend to demoralize the profession by forcing its members into unseemly rivalry, which would tend to enlarge the opportunity of the least scrupulous..." Sounds sensible? Not to the Federal Trade Commission, which ruled to abolish all such state initiatives.

HMOs and other similar prepaid plans are difficult to assess or place into a neat category. Remember, they contract to provide certain services at a fixed fee. The more patients the provider of those services can squeeze into a time slot, the better for them, but the worse for you. Rarely is there a freedom of choice option for you to pick the professional of your preference. This raises the competence question. You might assume that the HMO does your work in finding very qualified people. Not so. Often it comes down to who is willing to serve patients at the fees set by the HMO. (As the astronaut said before blasting off: "I try not to think that the rocket was built by the lowest bidder.")

If you are enrolled in a plan through your employer, you might try it out, but don't be surprised if the care is minimal and indifferent. Some optical chains have gotten into the HMO business by hardly charging the insuring provider for the cursory exams, then more than making it up through selling glasses and contact lenses. Deception might be too strong a word for this practice, but it's not far off.

With the knowledge you gain from this book, you will avoid all these pitfalls. When you find an optometrist you can feel comfortable with, stay with him or her. Over the years the doctor will become familiar with your eyes and vision, making any unusual changes readily apparent.

There's one more thing you can do—tell your friends about your optometrist so they won't have to go through the same search you did.

11

The Vision Examination:
What It Must Include

W e assume you are sensible enough to have your eyes examined on a regular basis, or perhaps you wait until you have an eye or vision problem. Either way, when you replace the phone after making an appointment, do you have some concept of what the examination should include? If it's your first examination, probably not. Even if you are an old hand at it, you may only have a general idea of what goes on. For your own welfare, you should really know more.

The optometrist's ability to diagnose your problem is based primarily on an extensive vision examination coupled with professional training and experience. Accordingly, the examination must cover a wide range of tests. If it doesn't, the diagnosis and your prescription/treatment can be incorrect.

Let's spell out the general examination so you'll be able to judge for yourself whether you are being properly cared for. We will describe what we consider to be the minimum tests and procedures. (Sometimes more are called for.) The exact order is not significant, but most doctors follow the sequence we will outline.

CASE HISTORY: You will be asked a lot of questions, the key one being, "What is your visual complaint?", or words to that effect. We also want to know when your problem started, how often and when it occurs, its severity, and what you've been doing to get relief. Some of these questions may seem irrelevant, but they give the experienced doctor some big clues toward a diagnosis.

When we ask about your occupation, we are not just being idly curious. You use your eyes quite differently as an accountant, a crane operator, a painter, or an auto mechanic. Your problem and symptoms might easily be tied in with your occupation (or hobby). Furthermore, the final prescription must take your job (hobby) into consideration.

"How is your general health?" and "Are you receiving any medical care or taking any medication?" must be answered fully and carefully since many ailments can affect the eyes. Diabetes is a prominent example; it can cause your sight to fluctuate. Please remember to mention all medications you are taking. It's best to prepare a list at home with all the names and dosages. Many drugs have side reactions which affect the eyes, ranging from mild lid swelling to serious retinal complications.

SCREENING TESTS: The objective is to find out how your eyes habitually perform in everyday life. The functions which should be measured are:
1. The sight in each eye at far and near, both with and without your current glasses.
2. Your color perception.
3. How well your eyes work together at far and near.
4. Whether there is intermittent suppression of either eye.
5. Your depth perception.
6. Whether the eyes move freely and accurately in all direction.

HEALTH: The health of your eyes is the concern of the next series of tests. First, the lids and surface parts of the eyes are inspected for any sign of disease or injury. A simple but vital test is to check the reaction of your pupils to light. You know that your pupils constrict in the presence of light, but did you know that if they do so unequally/sluggishly, or not at all, it may be the first symptoms of a disease or neurological disorder? Some drugs will also alter the pupil reaction.

To examine the front parts of the eyes, a slit lamp biomicroscope is used. It sounds fearful, but the instrument merely focuses a light beam onto the eye and magnifies the view of the anterior parts anywhere from about 10 to 50 times. The gradual progression of cataracts is monitored in this way. The slit lamp is also suitable for estimating the depth of the anterior chamber (a factor in glaucoma).

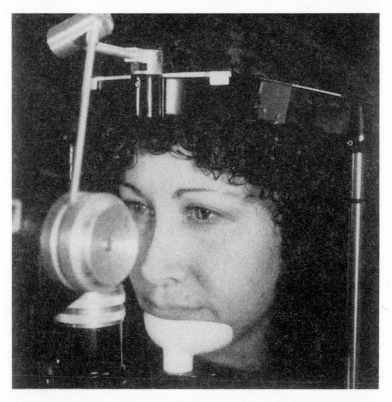

This patient is being examined with a biomicroscope or slit lamp which provides a highly magnified view of the anterior parts of the eye.

The optometrist will then turn his or her attention to examining the inside of the eyes with an ophthalmoscope. This instrument (there are many variations) lights up the inside of the eye and enlarges the image. Before doing this, the doctor may instill mydriatic drops into your eyes. The purpose of the drops is to dilate, enlarge the pupil for a better view, especially of the peripheral areas of the retina. The most commonly used drops dilate the pupil in about 20 to 30 minutes.

Inside the eye, we examine the retina, arteries, veins, and the optic nerve disc. Since the inside of the eye is the only place in the body where blood vessels can be seen in their natural state, it's an ideal opportunity to spot the first signs of hardening of the arteries, etc. We also look for, or rule out, specific eye diseases and abnormalities.

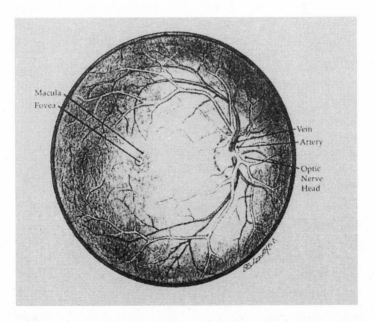

View of a normal retina of the right eye as seen through the pupil with an ophthalmoscope. Remember that this is a flat representation of a curved surface.

Notice the entrance of the optic nerve; the extensive branching of blood vessels across the retinal surface; and the scarcity of these blood vessels at the macula.

The test for fluid pressure inside the eye (so-called glaucoma test) can be done at this point or any other time. There are several methods, none of which should cause discomfort.

REFRACTION: (Note: if the eyes are to be dilated, this step should precede dilation.) Assuming that your eyes are healthy, the optometrist will assess their refractive condition which means that lenses are used to determine if you are nearsighted, farsighted, have astigmatism, or a combination of these. First, it's done objectively by directing your gaze at a distant target while a retinoscope light is focused into your eyes. (There are also automated instruments which can supply this information.) These results are refined subjectively with the familiar "Which is better?" coming into play. Some patients are very concerned about giving a wrong answer. Remember two things: 1. All the answers are double checked; 2. Sometimes the two views are, indeed, similar. If you do make a mistake it should not interfere with your final prescription.

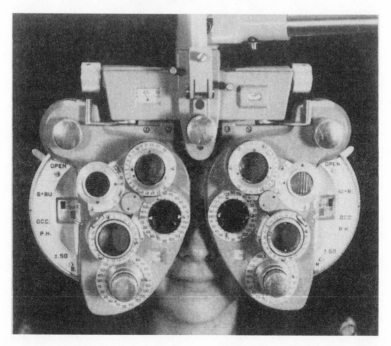

The phoropter is a convenient way to test vision. It embodies lenses and prisms making billions of combinations possible.

The refraction findings will be verified by using either a red and green line of letters or with polarizing filters.

In some circumstances and for specific individuals, a drop or two of a cycloplegic drug will be put into the eyes before the refraction. The aim is to paralyze the muscles that activate accommodation (focusing). Children represent the largest group for the use of cycloplegics. What are some of the common reasons for using those drops? Crossed eyes; suspected dormant hyperopia; suspected pseudomyopia (focusing muscles' spasm induces nearsightedness); sight not fully correctable to 20/20.

BINOCULARITY: Once your sight has been corrected, we want to know how your two eyes will work together with the intended corrective lenses. We will simulate seeing conditions you might encounter out in the everyday world, then measure the limits of your eyes to turn inward and outward, the flexibility of your focusing system, and your reserve capacity to avoid fatigue. What is the practical application of all this?

If you drive a bus, we want to know if you can maintain clear, comfortable vision hour after hour. If you are a lawyer, can you keep the small print from running together and/or blurring? If you are a student, can you easily change focus from the chalkboard to the reading material on your desk without tiring?

SUMMARY: The total examination can easily run to fifty or more individual items. The day is long since gone when all you had to do was read a few letters on a wall chart. That might have been adequate in the horse and buggy age, but it's completely outdated in our modern, complex society. If your examination is not as all-inclusive as we outlined, you are being taken for a ride in that buggy.

12

Special Tests
and Conditions

Occasionally, the routine examination will reveal or hint at some problem that requires further testing, or the patient may complain of one of the conditions we'll discuss. They should be investigated by the optometrist for possible referral to another medical specialist for a more definite diagnosis and/or treatment.

The Dry Eye

The normal eye is kept moist by a thin film of tears on its surface. This three-layer film is critically important for maintaining the function and health of the cornea. Since the cornea doesn't have a direct blood supply, the surface cells must maintain metabolism by getting oxygen and nutrients, then getting rid of waste products by way of the tear supply. (A complete lack of tears would cause the transparent cornea to become opaque with resulting blindness.) With each blink, the components of the tears, produced by the lacrimal gland and other glands in the lid, are spread across the cornea. If the tear production is reduced for any of a variety of reasons, you will suffer from hot, dry, burning eyes.

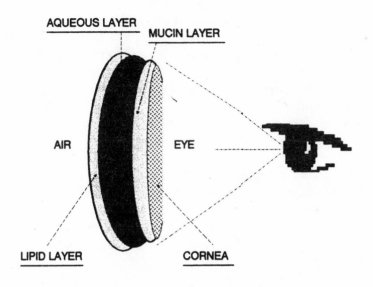

An enlargement of a tiny section of the front of the cornea showing, diagramatically, the three layers of the tear film. The mucin layer controls the amount of corneal wetting. The aqueous layer is the main watery reservoir. The surface lipid retards evaporation to the air.

This condition seems to be becoming more prevalent, so we'll go into more detail. The tear film is made up of three layers. The outer layer, composed of lipids (oily compounds), keeps the middle watery, aqueous layer from evaporating too rapidly. The inner layer of mucin controls the amount of water in contact with the cornea. When the watery layer evaporates too quickly, it leaves a higher salt concentration to irritate and burn the eyes.

For many people, the symptoms will appear during cold weather when the air is dry and further dried by indoor heating systems. During the summer, air conditioning could be the culprit. Other environmental factors such as dry climates, smoky rooms, wind and smog affect many individuals. The cause could be medication you are taking. Antihistamines and decongestants dry not only the mucous membranes of your nose but also dry your eyes. Some other medication examples which reduce the production of aqueous: diazepam (anti-anxiety), chlorpromazine (diabetic control), and atenolol (for hypertension). Tear production often naturally diminishes with the aging process. A disease such as Sjogren's syndrome, a systemic disorder often accompanying rheumatoid arthritis, will dry the eyes as well as the mouth.

Eye dryness is a frequent problem for people who wear contact lenses, especially soft, extended wear lenses. (See Guide to Successful Wear.)

There are a number of tests which can be used to quantify the problem. A common one is to instill a few drops of fluorescein to measure the tear break-up time, that is, how long it takes for the surface of the tears to evaporate. Another test makes use of Rose Bengal stain which selectively marks dry, dead cells. Neither test causes discomfort to the patient.

A dry eye can also ensue if the tear production is normal, but the blink reflex is missing or incomplete. There is an uncommon condition wherein the patient does not fully close his/her eyes during sleep. Injuries or burns to the lids can also forestall complete blinking. The exposed cornea can dry with serious consequences.

Mild cases of dry eyes can be eased with artificial tears or ointments. Severe cases may require sealing off the drainage tube in the lower lid to preserve what little moisture is available, or fitting a soft, therapeutic contact lens on the eye to protect the cornea.

The Wet Eye

This would seem to be the opposite of the dry eye, but in reality, sometimes is a reaction to the dry eye. Older people are commonly the victims, and the doctor must differentiate between an eye "feeling" wet vs. tears actually running down the cheeks. (See Chapter 34, Vision of the Aging.) To determine if a clogged drainage system is at fault, a few drops of fluorescein dye are put into the eye. After a minute or two, the patient blows his/her nose and the tissue is checked for fluorescein. A clogged drainage tube can be probed open fairly easily.

Loss of Corneal Sensitivity

The next time you get a piece of dust in your eye don't complain about the pain and buckets of tears. Be thankful that your system is working as it should. The pain, of course, is a warning that something is damaging the cornea; the profuse tearing is an attempt to wash the offending object away.

In some rare instances, the cornea may lose its sensitivity. If you can't feel foreign matter rubbing the cornea, serious eye damage can result. It's quite easy to test for sensitivity with an instrument or a thin wisp of cotton. Total lack of sensitivity indicates a serious neurological problem. This should not be confused with the gradual diminishing sensitivity of aging.

Bulging or Protruding Eyes

We are not referring to people with naturally large eyes such as very nearsighted individuals, but when one or both eyes give the appearance of becoming larger. It doesn't really mean that the eyes are getting bigger, but rather that they have started to protrude. If both eyes become more prominent,—"frog-eyed" look—chances are an overactive thyroid is responsible. When only one eye protrudes, the chief causes are hemorrhages, inflammation, or tumors which must be quickly dealt with. Often the protrusions are tenuous, and instruments must be used to carefully compare the two eyes.

Double Vision

If you have ever experienced double vision when you are tired, after taking medication, or after drinking too much alcohol, you know how very disturbing it can be. Sudden double vision without any apparent cause is very frightening. No matter what the reason, it attests that the two eyes are not pointing at the same spot.

In the case of fatigue or drugs (including alcohol), there is a temporary interruption with the brain's ability to control and coordinate the eye muscles. Getting sufficient rest or eliminating the offending chemical is usually all that's needed.

A more serious matter is double vision which occurs abruptly and is present all the time. The typical culprit is a small stroke or hemorrhage; less likely is a brain tumor. In most instances, proper treatment of the underlying cause may slowly restore single vision. As a temporary measure, special prism glasses can keep the double vision under control.

The Field of Vision

Normal vision is made up of two integrated systems—accurate, sharp sight when looking directly at an object coupled with a general awareness of the scene around you. To get the idea, do this simple experiment: Look straight ahead, hold your arms out at shoulder level and wriggle your fingers. With good peripheral vision you should be aware of the motion of your fingers. (This also illustrates that at the extreme edges of your field of vision, the main attention-getter is motion.)

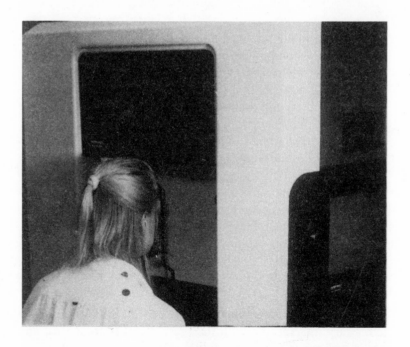

A field of vision testing instrument. The patient fixates a central target with one eye and responds to flashing and/or moving spots of light. An internal computer will analyze and provide a printed copy of the field of view.

If you lose either the central vision or the peripheral vision, you can be considered legally blind. You would suppose that having nice, clear central sight would be adequate, but it just isn't by itself. Why not? Roll two sheets of paper into small tubes, hold them up against your eyes and look through them. You can definitely watch TV and reading can be mastered, but try walking around in unfamiliar surroundings or descending a flight of stairs. Driving an automobile with any degree of safety would be impossible. Conversely, if your central sight is lost, you can walk around, but you would not be able to read or easily recognize people's faces.

There are many diseases which can decimate either the central or peripheral vision. Glaucoma is the classical example of one that gradually shrinks the peripheral vision until, in the final stage, only the narrow central sight remains.

Rather than the entire peripheral view being lost, it's more likely that a section or portion is missing. Usually, you won't even be aware of it because the blank area is filled in by the sight of the other eye. However, if the loss is to the outside or downward, and cannot be filled in, you may find yourself bumping into objects. These sector field losses can be caused by aneurisms, hemorrhages, tumors, etc.

The testing is generally done with computerized instruments which flash tiny spots of light against a blank background. The location, size and density of the missing area is plotted and recorded for analysis.

Amsler Grid

As the name implies, a grid of fine lines is used to detect subtle changes and distortions in the perceived view. While staring, with one eye at a time, at the central fixation dot, some portion of the lines may be seen to be missing or not perfectly straight. Retinal swelling, hemorrhages and certain diseases are the cause. Often, a patient will be given an Amsler grid to keep at home to monitor changes. (See page 70.)

Contrast Sensitivity

The ability to see an object in dim light or to detect an object against a background of almost similar shading, depends on a person's sensitivity to discern small differences in contrast.

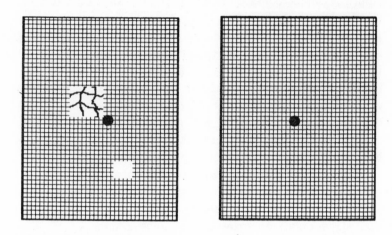

AMSLER GRID: *One eye is covered. The uncovered eye stares at the central fixation dot. All the lines should appear even and straight as on the left. Possible defects such as missing areas or distorted areas are illustrated on the right.*

The visual system has several subsystems (channels) each best tuned in to a particular level of contrast. The normal visual acuity test (20/40, 20/20, etc.) uses high contrast letters and is relatively insensitive for revealing any problems with the lower contrast channels. It's of interest because, after all, most of our general seeing is not concerned with reading black letters on a white background at 20 feet.

There are normal variations among individuals, but aging, eye diseases, diseases affecting the visual system, amblyopia and the use of certain medications can have negative consequences.

Your contrast sensitivity can be screened with a test that takes only a few minutes. The test is also useful in predicting improvement with a prescription change or a tinted lens, and it can alert the doctor to avoid a change or tint which could worsen the problem.

Extensive Color Testing

Color vision is routinely screened during the regular examination to detect any gross color deficiencies. For occupations requiring an excellent "color sense" such as printer, art director, stage-scenery designer, cloth dyer, etc., or for the detection of an early stage of a disease, more extensive color tests are administered. One such test requires arranging a series of round, colored discs in the correct sequence of hues. The most sophisticated color test, the anomaloscope, used mostly in research, challenges the person to mix primary green and red light sources together to match a standard yellow light.

Electrodiagnostic Tests

Very sensitive instruments can detect and measure the electrical nerve impulses which are generated in the eye and travel through the optic nerve to the brain. Similar in operation to an electrocardiogram, an electroretinogram (ERG) can provide practical information about the functioning of the retina in patients with acquired or inherited retinal disorders.

The more comprehensive visual evoked response (VER) test will measure the electrical activity along the visual pathway all the way to the visual cortex of the brain. Electrodes are attached to specific spots on the head, but there is no discomfort. The VER makes it possible to differentiate the vision in each eye, assess the potential visual acuity, and detect amblyopia objectively. It can be extremely useful with young children or retarded adults whose subjective responses could be unreliable or difficult to obtain.

Ultrasonography, Echography

When the inside of the eye cannot be clearly viewed because of a hemorrhage, cloudy fluid or a cataract, ultrasonography is employed to "see" what's inside. The technique generates sound waves and measures the returning echoes to harmlessly probe the eye and surrounding tissue for fractures, tumors, detachments, foreign bodies, etc. A very common use for ultrasonography is to measure the size and location of the eye's structures prior to cataract surgery to calculate the needed power of the lens to be implanted.

Fluorescein Angiography

This is an invasive test to assess the blood circulation in the retina and choroid at the back of the eye, or to verify the presence of a tumor. Fluorescein, a dye which glows in ultraviolet light, is injected into a vein and quickly circulates into the retinal vessels. Photographs taken every few seconds through a cobalt blue filter can pinpoint leaking, obstructed and/or new blood vessels. Because of a small but serious health-risk factor from the injected fluorescein, this procedure is used if the information cannot be gained in any other manner.

Gonioscopy

A gonioscope is essentially a contact lens fitted with tiny mirrors to view the angle opening between the cornea and iris inside the eye. The information gained can differentiate between open or closed angle glaucoma; inspect for tumors and lesions; recognize injury induced tears; evaluate effectiveness of laser treatments.

Interferometry

When a dense cataract is present, it is very important to estimate what degree of vision will be available after the cataract is removed. Since the view and inspection of the back of the eye is blocked by the cataract, the doctor may be unaware that retinal disease may also be present. If there is, removing the cataract will leave the person disappointed in the scantiness of sight improvement.

The interferometer focuses an intense, coherent source of regular or laser light into the eye to establish an approximate idea of the reclaimable vision. The instrument is also practical for predicting the eventual sight attainable after treatment for amblyopia.

Glare Tester

Cataracts or other opacities in the eye will often cause increased sensitivity to glare because they scatter the incoming light. If the glare source is bright enough it will functionally reduce your sight. For instance, a person may see 20/30 in normal illumination, but barely see 20/200 in very bright light.

A glare testing instrument can document the levels of glare which creates a disability, and can help determine if tints applied to the glasses can be beneficial in minimizing the effects. Another use for the instrument is to measure the time it takes to recover sight after the retina is dazzled with very bright light. This mimics entering a darkened area after exposure to sunlight, or being "blinded" by oncoming headlights in night driving. While the glare-recovery time normally increases with age, very slow recovery can also be caused by disease or vitamin deficiency.

Radiology, CT-Scan, MRI

Suspected fractures of any of the bones making up the eye socket will require X-ray pictures to identify the breaks. For complicated fractures with muscle entrapment, to localize foreign bodies, and investigate for suspected tumors, Computed Tomography (CT-SCAN) makes diagnosis easier. Magnetic Resonance Imaging (MRI) is more useful to differentiate between diseases of soft tissues, though it should not be employed when a metallic foreign body is present.

Cell Counts

The inner layer of the cornea, the endothelium, plays a crucial role in maintaining the transparency and health of the cornea. Unlike the surface epithelial layer, the endothelium doesn't grow new cells to replace damaged ones. The remaining cells enlarge to fill in the spaces. (Long term contact lens wear seems to be implicated with changes in the cell shapes.)

Before cataract removal or corneal surgery, an instrument is often used to estimate the number and determine the condition of the cells. Since many are lost during surgery, the information helps assess the risk and success of the surgical procedure.

Pachometry

There are instances when it is important to know the thickness of the cornea and the depth of the anterior chamber of the eye. The pachometer, an instrument attached onto the biomicroscope (slit lamp) will accomplish this. A very useful application is to measure corneal swelling or thickening after contact lenses are worn for an extended time.

Ophthalmodynamometer

An instrument designed specifically to measure the systolic and diastolic blood pressure of arterioretinal vessels. It will often detect increasing intracranial pressure before other symptoms appear. (This instrument is giving way to more sophisticated methods.)

IV

All About Glasses

13

How Do Glasses Work?

You were probably not too thrilled the first time you were told you needed glasses, but as long as you must wear them, why not learn how they work? Obviously, glasses are made up of lenses and a frame. The frame can be made of plastic, metal, or a combination of the two; its function is to keep the lenses positioned in front of your eyes. The part that sits on the bridge of your nose is called, quite logically, the "bridge," and the handles which fit on your ears are called "temples." Within certain limitations which will be described in later chapters, you can have free reign in your choice of frame styles and colors. It's the lenses, of course, which make the whole contraption so useful.

Basically, what is a lens? It doesn't have to be made out of glass or plastic to do its job. The only requirement is that it be transparent and capable of bending—refracting—light rays in a predetermined way. You could, if you put your mind to it, make a lens out of ice or gelatin and fulfill the basic requirement. It would make an interesting science fair project, but pretty strange glasses. No, we need something more durable.

Whether glass or plastic is used, it must be manufactured totally free of tiny air bubbles, striations, and distortions; it requires very exacting techniques. There are plenty of rejects and "seconds" in lenses which, unfortunately, find their way to unscrupulous operators and so-called "bargain" houses.

The lens power is measured in units called diopters which are based on the extent to which the light rays passing through the lens will be bent. As the power of the lens increases, so does the thickness. Three types of lenses are commonly used to correct vision problems—convex, concave, and cylindrical.

The convex lens is thicker in the center that at the edges, and gathers light rays together towards a point. Remember when you were a kid and used a magnifying lens to focus the sun's rays on a piece of paper in order to start it burning? That was a convex lens. It is used in glasses for the farsighted eye which cannot bend the light rays as mush as they should. If the eye is 2 diopters farsighted, a 2 diopter convex lens will compensate for it. It is also commonly used in reading glasses.

The concave lens is thinner at the center than at the edges, and spreads light rays apart. You could not use this lens to focus the sun's rays, because it never forms a real image anywhere. (The explanation involves physics—just take our word for it.) By putting this lens in front of the nearsighted eye, we can reduce the overall power to put the image neatly on the retina. A 1 diopter concave lens will correct 1 diopter of nearsightedness.

The cylindrical lens is shaped like a section of an auto tire, curved more in one direction than the other. It's very difficult to ascertain the direction of the curve by simply looking at your glasses. Sometimes you can recognize it this way: Hold the glasses about twenty inches in front of you and sight a straight line or edge through the lens. Slowly rotate the glasses clockwise and then counterclockwise. If the line tilts with or against the rotation of the glasses, it's a cylindrical lens and you have astigmatism. This type of lens must be carefully aligned in front of the eyes with an exact up and down orientation. Most often a cylindrical lens will be part of the prescription with a convex or concave lens.

Would you like to learn how to read a prescription for eyeglasses? A convex lens (for the farsighted eye) is written with a plus (+) symbol. A concave lens (for the nearsighted eye) is written with a minus (-) sign. If the prescription calls for a +2.00, it's a 2 diopter lens for a farsighted eye, or it could be a 2 diopter reading lens for a presbyopic eye. A -2.50 is a 2 1/2 diopter lens for a nearsighted eye. The higher the number the stronger the lens.

For an eye with astigmatism, the prescription might look like this:

$$-2.50 \ -1.00 \ \text{axis} \ 45$$

This is 2 1/2 diopters of nearsightedness with 1 diopter of astigmatism. The axis indicates the orientation of the cylindrical part of the lens. It's based on the degrees of a protractor—180 is the horizontal, 90 the vertical meridians. The axis can be anywhere from 1 to 180.

A bifocal prescription will have additional numbers to indicate the strength of the reading part of the lens.

$$+1.75 \ -0.25 \ \text{axis} \ 95$$
$$\text{add} \ +1.50$$

This is 1 3/4 diopters of farsightedness with 1/4 diopter of astigmatism and an additional 1 1/2 diopters of power for reading.

Sometimes a prism effect has to be incorporated into the prescription to deviate the light rays in a desired way.

$$-3.25 \ -0.75 \ \text{axis} \ 70 \ 2^{\Delta} \ \text{IN}$$

The little triangular figure designates a prism and in this case the direction of the base is inward, though it could be out, up or down.

You need one more piece of information in order to read your RX—knowing which numbers are for which eye. The right eye is designated O.D. for the Latin oculus dexter; the left eye is O.S. for oculus sinister. O.U. is oculus uterque, both eyes.

You may still not be thrilled about having to wear glasses, but at least you now know what you're wearing.

14

Getting Used To Your Glasses

When you get glasses for the first time, or when there is a change in your prescription, it will upset your visual world. Certainly you can expect clearer sight and more comfortable vision, but along with that you will notice some strange side effects. Objects may appear larger or smaller, closer or farther, and familiar shapes may be deformed. Don't hit the panic button. These effects are only temporary and within a few days you should be completely unaware of them. But why the problem in the first place? There are several reasons.

Because of technical limitations, only the very center of the lens has the exact prescription your eye needs. When you look away from the center (and you do every time you move your eyes), you're actually looking through a slightly different prescription. This difference increases towards the edge of the lens and causes shapes and sizes to be distorted. The thicker the lens, the greater the distortion; the larger the lens, the more edge distortion. (The eye is increasingly farther from the lens margin.) In low power prescriptions, the warping of objects and space is manageable and you can adjust quickly. With high powers, the adjustment can be very difficult, and large size glasses should be avoided.

Another factor influencing your sight with glasses is the curvature of the lens surfaces. It is possible to produce lenses having the same prescription power but with a variety of curvatures. A lens can be made with one flat surface, two modest curves or nearly bulging. So what? The curvatures affect the image size and shape seen through that lens. For example, a concave lens for a nearsighted person will produce a larger image if made with a deep curve. If the prescription in your two eyes is quite different, it is no easy matter to select matching curvatures.

Has it ever happened to you that two supposedly identical pairs of glasses don't feel the same? It could be that they were made with lenses of dissimilar curvatures.

If you are nearsighted and put glasses on for the first time, the world will look clearer but smaller. Since the brain uses size as one judgment of distances (small objects are assumed to be farther away), you will tend to think you are more remote from things than you really are. You may spill a cup of coffee when you reach for it because it's closer than you visualize.

If you are farsighted, the opposite will happen. Objects will appear clearer but larger. So, you will judge things to be closer and when you reach for a doorknob you may come up short. Over the span of a few days, the brain will recalculate object/distance relationships and you will regain your familiar distance judgement.

These annoyances are minor compared to the first-time correction for astigmatism. Objects will be tilted and curved; your entire perspective will be in shambles. (You'll appreciate what fictional Alice experienced.) Be courageous—as confusing as things may be, they will slowly reassemble into a "normal" looking world within a few days.

Scientific and technical advancements in lens materials now makes it possible to produce thin, lightweight lenses out of high-index resins. The higher the index of refraction of a lens material, the more prescription power can be squeezed into a given area. The result is a dramatic, cosmetic improvement in the way the finished glasses look. However, because the prescription power is intensified, moving the eyes off the lens center will cause a quicker change in effective strength. It will take a little longer to adapt to glasses with these materials, but it's well worth it.

A seemingly minor matter such as the distance between the lens and your eye will effect the power and image size. If you are farsighted and the glasses slip down your nose, the effective power and image size are increased. If you are nearsighted and wear your glasses at the end of your nose, the effective power is reduced. The exact amount will vary with the length of your nose and the prescription.

All the annoying symptoms are aggravated proportionally with high power prescriptions. The very nearsighted person also has to contend with unsightly, thick, light-reflecting edges on the lenses. While these can be reduced with the high-index lenses, a further improvement can be made by "rolling" the edges and tinting the lens. A better way is to choose a smaller frame because the edge thickness increases sharply with increased lens size.

A very farsighted person need not be concerned with a thick edge, but the eyes exhibit an enlarged "bug-eyed" look from the bulky center thickness. This can largely be overcome with special high-index materials which are designed with unique curvatures to flatten the center bulge. Of course, the adaptation time will be longer.

Some people are bothered by reflections from the surfaces of the lenses, especially at night. You should have little trouble learning to ignore them, but if desired, the reflections can be mostly eliminated with a multilayered, anti-reflective coating on the surfaces.

To get the best vision, the centers of the lenses must be positioned directly in front of your pupils. Rarely does the frame size exactly match this position. Therefore, the lenses must be offset to compensate for the actual eye placement. If this is not done, it can disturb your eye movements and focusing.

For all these reasons, it should be apparent that the making of glasses must not be a haphazard procedure. The measuring,

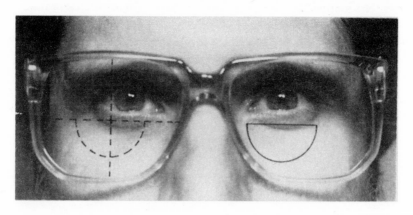

When glasses are fitted, the eyes must look through the optical center of the lenses for maximum sight and comfort.

In most cases, as is shown here, the position of the eyes do not match the actual center of the lens (seen on the left). On the right is a properly centered bifocal lens.

fitting and aligning of the glasses has to be done accurately and knowledgeably. For your own good, the optometrist should oversee the entire process.

Care and Handling

There are a number of things you should do to keep the glasses in good condition. When you put them on or take them off, use both hands and hold them by the temples (ear pieces). Try not to pull the temples outward. Women are especially guilty of this while trying to protect a hairdo.

Never lay the glasses on any surface with the lenses down. Doing this repeatedly will breed scratches. Instead, lay them on the temples or put them into the case.

Dirt can easily accumulate around the rims between the frame and lens edge. It's easy to remove with an old, soft toothbrush and warm, soapy water.

With plastic lenses, even "scratch resistant" types, always wash the dirt and grit off before wiping gently with a soft cloth or tissue. If you have no immediate access to water, rather than wiping them when dry, just blow the dust off.

No matter how careful you are, with occasional bumping and handling, the frame may become crooked and misaligned. You should return for proper frame adjustment to avoid discomfort and visual disturbances. The original fee for the glasses generally includes this service.

15

Bifocals and Multifocals

When the doctor told you that you needed bifocals, you may have protested (verbally or only mentally) that you weren't that old. Actually, you probably weren't, even though a few grey hairs may have started to show up here and there. The average person begins to need bifocals in their 40s, and then only if he or she does reading or close work. Five hundred years ago when most people where illiterate and/or occupied with farming, bifocals were not necessary. (The life span was much shorter, too.) Today, they are almost indispensable.

A simple way to describe a bifocal is to say that it has two prescriptions combined into one lens. A trifocal has three prescriptions combined into one lens; a progressive bifocal has a "continuous" number.

That old kite flyer, Benjamin Franklin, came up with the idea for the bifocal in the 18th century. He found it very bothersome to switch back and forth from his distance glasses to his reading glasses all day long. His clever solution was to cut each set of lenses into half moons (lenses were perfectly round in those days), and put them together in one frame. The top half was for his distance prescription and the bottom half his reading lenses.

No matter what form or shape modern bifocals have, they are essentially two pairs of glasses put together. As in Franklin's case, the most common reason for bifocals is presbyopia—when the eyes can no longer easily focus at near small objects. If you wear only reading glasses distance vision is blurred and they have to be removed to see far away. If you also need glasses for distance seeing, then you are in Ben's predicament. By placing the reading prescription in only the lower part of the lens, there is little interference with normal distance seeing.

There are many variations in design of the modern bifocal lens. The particular one chosen for you must depend on your prescription, occupation, life style, etc. The reading segment can be any size, from very small to very large; its top edge can be flat, round or oval; it can be positioned high or low in the frame. The possible combinations can run into the hundreds.

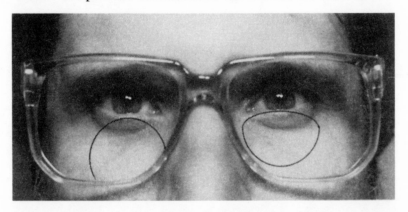

Left: Round bifocal. Right: Oval top bifocal.

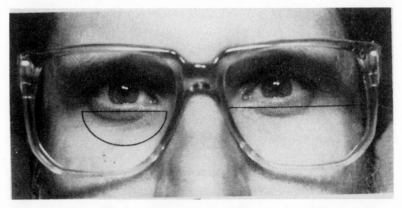

Left: Flat top bifocal. Right: Executive bifocal.

What are some of the factors in choosing a bifocal? How you use them is the main consideration. Here are two extreme examples: A symphony musician must read the music at about twenty-four inches and also occasionally glance at the conductor thirty feet away for the tempo. This person needs a bifocal with a large reading area and just a small distance portion at the top. On the other hand, a golfer wants a large distance portion with just a tiny reading spot to write on the score card. The reading position must be very low in the frame so it's out of the line of sight when the golfer addresses the ball.

Each patient must have the bifocals designed for his or her particular use. Many times it's impossible to design an "all purpose" bifocal for all activities. This is quite obvious when you consider that the musician could also be an avid golfer. You can't expect to use the same bifocals for all occasions, any more than you would wear a suit of armor on the golf course.

The prescription strength of the reading portion can be made, within reason, for the distance at which you will use it. A carpenter working at arm's length wants to see clearly at about twenty-four inches; someone working a sewing machine would prefer to see clearly at about fifteen inches. That doesn't mean you are limited to exactly twenty-four and fifteen inches respectively. Depending on your age, there is a latitude of clear vision both closer and behind these distances.

Certain occupations require rather unusual lenses. For instance, a pharmacist has to be able to read labels on shelves well above eye level as well as normal reading material. A double bifocal, with a reading segment at the top and bottom serves this purpose. An electrician doing overhead wiring would also benefit from this arrangement.

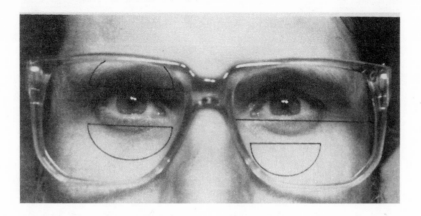

Left: Double flat top. Right: Occupational trifocal.

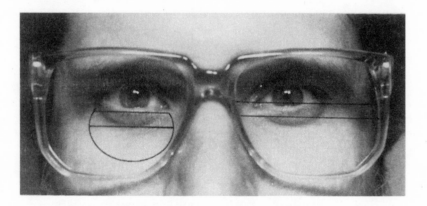

Left: Flat top trifocal. Right: Executive trifocal.

Trifocals are three pairs of glasses in one. Why would any-one need three different prescriptions? As you get older and the eye's focusing flexibility dwindles, you may not be able to see clearly at all distances with a bifocal. The distance pre-scription at the top of the lens will let you see distinctly from about four feet all the way out to the stars; the reading segment will let you see up close. This leaves an area from about twenty inches to three feet which will be fuzzy. If you need or desire clear vision at that distance, the in-between segment of the tri-focal will supply it. A typical user would be a computer operator who would use the mid-range portion to read the characters on the video screen.

In normal bifocals or trifocals there is an abrupt change in the prescription from one section to the next. One class of lens designs gaining in popularity has a continuously changing prescription from the distance to the reading power. These are called progressive addition lenses. Theoretically, all seeing is clear if you look through the appropriate part of the lens. In practice, it takes quite a bit of adaptation because the size of the intermediate and reading zones are rather small. Also, there are distortions at the edges of these zones. Most people do adapt within about a week and are quite pleased with the results. These multifocals do away with the normally visible dividing lines and are called "invisible". They are, therefore, more acceptable cosmetically.

When you get your first bifocals, you'll have to develop new seeing habits combined with different patterns of head and eye movement relationships. For one thing, when walking down stairs, don't just lower your eyes. If you do, you'll be looking through the reading segment and the steps will be blurry. Just lower your chin to look through the upper section and the stairs will be clear. Another common problem for beginning bifocal wearers is trying to read a notice on a bulletin board. Simply raise your chin until the reading section is in position.

Most people learn to use bifocals fairly rapidly, and within a week or ten days have everything mastered. A few people just never seem to be able to get the hang of it and must revert to using two pairs of glasses with its inherent nuisance. If you are one of these people, have the optometrist re-asses your vision needs. It's possible that you were trying to use the wrong type of bifocal for your particular needs.

16

Sunglasses and Tinted Lenses

Sunglasses are, of course, a type of tinted lenses. Because of their widespread and common use, we have given them top billing. You probably use sunglasses for relief from the intense glare of sunlight, but do you know what else you should be protecting yourself from?

The light with which our eyes see is only a fraction of the radiation given off by the sun. If you recall your physics, you know that the radiation extends from the minuscule gamma rays, beyond X-rays, ultraviolet, visible light, infrared and all the way to the very long radio waves. It is no coincidence that the visible light to which our eyes are sensitive is precisely that radiation which is reflected from solid objects such as trees, rocks, and people.

If you have ever idly wished you had Superman's X-ray vision, you would quickly change your mind the first time you were injured after walking into a brick wall which is transparent to X-rays. Note how many people are injured walking into plate glass doors which are transparent to visible light. Obviously, our visual system evolved to give us the most useful information about our surroundings.

Some of the radiation from the sun (or artificial sources) is harmful to our biological design. A critical point: to be harmful or have any effect at all, the radiation must be absorbed. No absorption, no effect. For example, radio waves pass through our bodies without being absorbed and without any apparent detrimental effect. On the other hand, X-rays are absorbed by certain tissues, are therefore dangerous, and must be shielded with lead (which absorbs them).

The two kinds of radiation we are normally exposed to and which may cause eye problems are the ultraviolet (UV) and the infrared (IR). Both are invisible as far as the eye is concerned but infrared can be sensed as heat by the skin. We have no sense organ to detect ultraviolet, but its absorption on the skin leads to suntan or sunburn. There is another distinction between these two radiations on biological tissues: UV effects are cumulative over time; IR is not. (The aging and cancer risk on the skin from UV is related to repeated exposures.)

Let's examine what these rays can do to your eyes. The UV is absorbed almost totally by the cornea, the balance by the lens inside the eye, with some reaching the retina. (Macular degeneration is suspected from UV absorbed by the retina.) Therefore, using the formula, absorption = effect, any dire consequences will be mainly on the cornea, then the lens. The surface layer of the cornea can blister and hurt much more than any sunburn you've ever had. This sometimes happens to people who thoughtlessly read under a sunlamp, forgetting that the UV is reflected off the paper onto the eyes. It's a very painful experience.

Chronic exposure to UV (and perhaps, IR) has been implicated with the development of cataracts in the lens of the eye.

The infrared (heat) rays are absorbed partly by the cornea, partly by the lens, but a good portion gets through to the retina. There is evidence that infrared rays cause burns on the delicate retinal tissue. That's the apparent scenario when you look at the sun during an eclipse. While the fiercely bright visible light is blocked, massive amounts of IR can enter the eye and focus on the retina. Depending on the duration and intensity, the retina may be burned, causing permanent scars and some loss of vision.

There are a host of commonly prescribed drugs which can make your eyes more photosensitive and susceptible to injury. These include: Allopurinol (for gout), Chlorpromazine (tranquilizer), Isotretinoin (acne therapy), and Tetracyclines (antibiotic.)

By now you should have the idea that sunglasses are more than just a fashion accessory. A point must be made about bright light itself. If you spend a day at the beach, for instance, without some type of glare protection, the photoreceptor pigment in the retina becomes bleached and your night vision will be poor. Older people must take even more precaution because the eye's ability to recover visual sensitivity after exposure to brightness is greatly reduced after age 40.

Non-Prescription Sunglasses

If you wear sunglasses and think you are protected, we have a surprise for you. There is no way for you to determine by either the color or the darkness whether they actually filter out the harmful rays. The color of the lens is not what counts, rather the chemical ingredient added to the glass to produce the color. For example, a dark green glass properly made will absorb virtually all the harmful rays; another green glass without the proper ingredients, will not. Worse than that, because the imitation lenses reduce the visible glare (nature's warning flag), it actually may be more harmful than not wearing colored lenses. (It's like the eclipse situation described before. The glare is blocked while the infrared passes through into your eyes.)

The confusion in the field of ready-made, so-called sunglasses is deplorable. You can find glasses with every conceivable color and degree of darkness promoted as sunglasses. Some of the worst junk is made for kids. Can you tell the good from the bad? It's very difficult. In the fifteen years since we called attention to this problem in our first edition, there has been improvement in the labeling as the public has been made more aware of the dangers of UV. At the very least, ultraviolet protection should be listed on the glasses. However, that does not address the problem of infrared or cheap and vision-distorting lenses.

One of our most frustrating experiences is standing in a variety store checkout line and watching people at a carousel of "sunglasses" and choosing one by the way it looks. Doing it that way may make you look "cool", but it may also "cook" your eyes.

The best all-around sunglasses contain properly made dark grey or dark green glass lenses. The "smoky" grey tint allows colors to be seen almost normally; the green filters out a bit more UV and IR. The choice is yours. Blue and yellow, regardless of how dark, are not good as sunglasses. However, yellow lenses may be used to increase visibility on a cloudy or hazy day. They enhance contrast by filtering out the somewhat scattered, out-of-focus blue light from the scene. Hunters, pilots, tennis players, etc., find them helpful for this purpose.

Polarizing sunglasses will significantly reduce glare coming off flat surfaces such as water, and are popular with fishermen. Their UV shielding is adequate but IR protection is poor.

There is a category of tinted glasses which are advertised as "blue blockers." Essentially, they filter out the UV and the blue end of the spectrum which is alongside the UV. Removing the blue light causes colors to appear false and is annoying to some individuals. More than just annoying, it is inappropriate for people who need good color discrimination and for those who have a color deficiency. The "sharpness of seeing" claim is for the same reason that yellow lenses "sharpen" vision. Along with the apparent clarity, you may experience errors in distance judgement - objects will appear closer. The quality and glare reduction in any particular pair are uncertain; also, there is no IR protection. All in all, there is no advantage to these orange-colored lenses over neutral tinted sunglasses. On the other hand, if you really like them and they have good UV filtering, you may choose to wear them.

Good sunglasses are not cheap. Conversely, spending a lot of money for a "designer" pair does not guarantee quality. Ideally, all sunglasses should have labels with transmission graphs as shown in the illustration. Then you could intelligently choose lenses for your exact need.

An example of how a transmission chart would look. The curves for three tinted materials have been plotted. Note that the green lens transmits about 50% of the green light, more than at any other wavelength, hence its green color; the PhotoGray lens transmits fairly evenly across blue, green, and red, hence the grey color. By looking at this type of chart, you can almost customize the tint to your special needs.

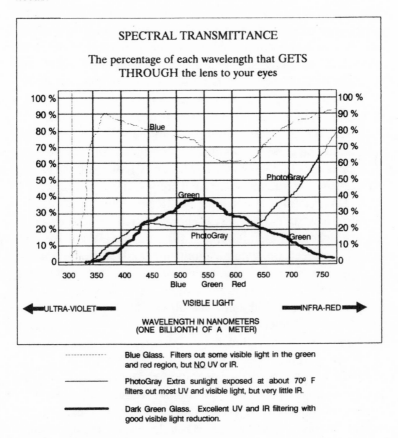

SPECTRAL TRANSMITTANCE

The percentage of each wavelength that GETS THROUGH the lens to your eyes

VISIBLE LIGHT

ULTRA-VIOLET   INFRA-RED

WAVELENGTH IN NANOMETERS
(ONE BILLIONTH OF A METER)

- - - - - - - - -   Blue Glass. Filters out some visible light in the green and red region, but NO UV or IR.

———————   PhotoGray Extra sunlight exposed at about 70º F filters out most UV and visible light, but very little IR.

████████   Dark Green Glass. Excellent UV and IR filtering with good visible light reduction.

Prescription Sunglasses

Now let's discuss prescription sunglasses which are made to the same Rx as your regular glasses. First of all, if you normally need to wear glasses you should also avail yourself of this convenience and protection. Granted there are clip-ons and slip-ins to cover your glasses, the results are just not as effective and they can also scratch your lenses. Prescription sunglasses can be made with glass or plastic lenses. As a general rule of thumb, plastic lenses have a better UV absorption characteristic, glass lenses can be made with more IR protection. The boundaries are not firm, however, and the best bet is to look at the transmission graphs or tell your optometrist what protection you need and want.

There are two ways to fabricate prescription sunglasses: (1) For glass lenses, the glass itself is colored before the prescription is ground into it; (2) For glass or plastic, the finished clear lens is chemically tinted to whatever hue is desired. The second method has the advantage of being evenly tinted regardless of lens thickness.

Included in the first groups, photochromic glass for lenses has been available for several decades. This material has microscopic silver crystals added into the molten glass mixture before it's fabricated into lenses. These crystals will darken when exposed to sunlight (mostly from the UV) and lighten when out of the sunlight. The darkening cycle intensity is a variable of several factors: temperature, lens thickness, the number of silver crystals, and the safety-hardening method. Odd as it may seem intuitively, the lenses darken much more in cool weather than on a hot day. Hence, they are acceptable for skiing and high altitudes (where more UV is present). However, they are poor for providing IR protection. They are also poor at darkening to a real sunglass when driving an automobile because the windshield blocks out most of the UV which normally darkens the lenses.

These photogray or photobrown glasses (there are differences in the tint and absorption action) which supposedly can be worn at all times have the limitation of not darkening enough in sunlight, darkening too much on a cloudy day, nor clearing completely at night. After a week or two, they retain a residual tint, even when you might want optimum light transmission. This can be a disturbing problem for older people whose eyes, with normal aging, require more light. (See The Vision of the Aging.) For young people, photochromic glasses might be suitable, but we do not recommend that choice as the only glasses for anyone over, say, 45.

To overcome the weight and safety factor of glass photochromic lenses, attempts have been made to somehow create plastic photo-reactive lenses. One method bonds a microscopic layer of material on the front surface of the lens which will darken and/or change colors in sunlight. They do provide fairly decent UV protection, but are even more inversely sensitive to temperature than the glass photochromics. Above 80°F they function poorly; approaching 100°F the color remains quite light. If the idea of a lens changing colors appeals to you, if the additional cost is no obstacle, and you don't mind the limitations, there is no harm in getting photo-reactive plastic eyeglasses.

Not to be outdone in reducing the weight of glass photochromics, the manufacturer has recently introduced a thinner, lighter-weight glass lens with a better darkening cycle. It is worth your consideration

Sunglasses at Night?

Never wear sunglasses when driving at night. While it may reduce the glare from oncoming headlights, it will also reduce your ability to see the road and potential hazards. On a dark night, it is estimated that sunglasses will reduce your seeing distance by one third which translates into one third less reaction time to avoid an accident.

Tinted Lenses and Coatings

It is technically possible to tint or coat the surface of a prescription lens with hundreds of hues as well as special materials to provide scratch resistance, glare reduction, to be anti-reflective, and cosmetically appealing. Many of these can be combined to individual specifications and needs.

Since the majority of prescription spectacles are made with plastic (CR-39) lenses, adding scratch-resistant surfaces might be high on your list of "musts." This is done by depositing a thin, clear film of quartz on the lenses. On the other hand, many of the new hi-index plastics are already provided with scratch resistant surfaces and even have a better UV filtering ability. (See Chapter 17, Shatter-Resistant Glass or Plastic Lenses.) Another useful addition is an anti-reflective (A/R) coating to reduce the often annoying spots of glimmering light reflected from the lens surface. A/R is comparable to the faint bluish coatings on quality camera and binocular lenses.

When thinking about lens colors and coatings, you should consider your occupation, hobbies and life-style. You can't expect one pair of glasses to do everything any more than you would expect your high-heel dress shoes to be suitable for golf, tennis and boating. The accompanying charts are good guidelines to the most frequent and useful tints. It is very important to understand that you can't tell a tint's absorption by its color. There are many manufacturers of coloring compounds and the quality varies. As we mentioned before, a transmission chart is the only way to be certain of what you're getting.

For some people, a gradient tint which is darker at the top of the lens and lightens towards the bottom, is beneficial. The original idea was born during World War II when pilots used gradient sunglasses. The dark upper halves blocked the glare from the sky, while the lower clear portion permitted reading the dim cockpit instruments. Unless you're a pilot, gradient sunglasses are not a great idea since in general use there is glare and radiation being reflected upward from sidewalks, sandy beaches, etc. However, lightly tint gradient lenses may be prescribed for office workers, for example, who work under bright overhead fluorescents.

Vision Enhancing Lenses

People with developing cataracts, macular and retinal degeneration and glaucoma may be particularly bothered by the glare created by shortwave blue light. Any tint which blocks the blue light is helpful in increasing contrast and visibility. Corning Glass Works has available a photochromic glass lens which not only removes the blue light but adjusts its darkness to suit the light conditions.

Speciality Lenses

Many industrial processes require tinted lenses to protect workers from specific harmful radiation. For example, glassblowers must use lenses that reduce the transmittance of the near infrared region because molten glass is very high in that output. There is also a special lens to provide protection from X-ray radiation. Industry management people are generally well aware of the potential hazards and every effort is made to protect the employees.

TINT REFERENCE GUIDE FOR SPECIFIC USES

WORK, HOBBY, INTERESTS	SUGGESTED COLOR AND/OR COATING
Boating / Sailing	Dark Green, Grey or Brown with added mirror coating.
Tennis	Amber or Gold/Yellow indoors or on cloudy days. Green or Grey on sunny
Skiing / Snowmobiling	Dark Green, Grey or Brown with added mirror coating and/or UV coating.
Racquetball	Amber or Gold/Yellow with anti-reflective coating.
Hunting	Gold/Yellow with anti-reflective coating on cludy days. Green or Grey in sunlight.
Sewing / Needlecraft	Light Rose, Brown, Pecan, etc. with anti-reflective coating.
Baseball, Football, Soccer, Field Hockey (Outdoor action sports)	Medium Green, Grey or Brown.
Fishing in bright sun	Dark Green, Grey or Brown with polarizing filter.
Night driving	Anti-reflective coating.
Beach vacation	Dark Green or Grey with UV and IR filter.
Computer screen	Light tint with anti-reflective coating.
Piloting	Dark Green or Grey Gradient with UV filter.
Golf	Green or Grey on sunny days. Amber or Gold/Yellow on cloudy days
Office work with bright overhead lighting.	Light to medium gradient tint in Rose, Brown, Pecan, etc.

SELECTION GUIDE TO TINTED GLASS LENSES

COLOR		PERCENTAGE OF ABSORPTION			USES
		UV	VISIBLE	IR	
CLEAR		7%	6%	7%	
PINK	Light	20%	15%	10%	Cuts glare from artificial lights. Modest
	Medium	45%	25-35%	10%	UV protection.
BLUE		95%	10%	12%	Cosmetic use only. NOT for sunlight.
YELLOW		65%	35%	10%	Increased visibility in haze or fog.
GREEN	Medium	90%	60%	90%	Good sunglasses.
	Dark	80%	80%	95%	Excellent sunglasses.
BROWN	Medium	90%	50%	60%	Good sunglasses.
	Dark	95%	75%	80%	Very good sunglasses.
GRAY	Medium	95%	60%	60%	Good sunglasses.
	Dark	95%	80%	70%	Excellent sunglasses.
PHOTO- CHROMIC	Light	80%	50%	40%	General wear, winter sports.
	Extra	85%	80%	35%	Sunglasses in cool climates.

These percentages are averages and may vary depending on the manufacturer. The absorption also depends on the thickness of the lens which is about 2 m.m. for these figures. Example: Dark green absorbs 95% of IR and only about 5% gets to your eyes.

17

Shatter-Resistant Glass or Plastic Lenses

ince January of 1972, federal law has required that lenses for glasses be made shatter resistant. Until then, a high proportion of eyeglasses were fabricated with glass lenses and breakage was fairly common. If the lens shattered while being worn, eye injuries could result. As written, the law specifies "shatter resistant"—resistant to shattering, not immune to shattering. They are neither safety lenses nor unbreakable, and should not be thought of in that way. The most descriptive term is "dress hardened", meaning impact resistant for everyday, general dress wear.

To be considered shatter resistant, the lens must be capable of withstanding the impact of a half ounce, 5/8th of an inch steel ball dropped onto the lens from a height of 50 inches. (For safety-in-industry use, the lens must withstand a heavier steel ball drop.) Ordinary glass lenses subjected to this test would shatter into tiny sharp fragments and could cause serious eye injury.

There are several ways to "harden" a glass lens to make it shatter resistant. One method is to heat the lens to a fairly high temperature and then quickly cool with a blast of cool air. A second method is to chemically harden the surfaces by immersing the lens in a hot chemical solution for hours. Finally, a glass lens can be made shatter resistant by laminating a thin sheet of plastic into the center like a slice of ham between slices of bread.

A drawback for the patient is that no matter which method is used, the lens must be thicker (a minimum of 2.2 millimeters for regular and 3 millimeters for industrial use) and consequently, heavier. The thicker lenses are cosmetically unwelcome and the added weight can be harsh on the bridge of the nose.

If you do wear such glasses, whether "dress hardened" or "safety hardened", inspect them regularly for scratches or tiny pits which will seriously compromise their resistance to breakage.

After 1972, the pendulum slowly began to swing towards the use of plastic lens materials, and today most glasses contain plastic lenses. There are many benefits. The nature of the material itself, a resin, makes it four times as shatter resistant as hardened glass. Even if a strong enough blow causes breakage, the pieces are not sharp and have little penetrating force. Not only is the lens quite safe, but it has the amazing ability to shed sparks from welding and grinding which would pit glass lenses.

Aside from the safety feature, there are a couple of nice bonuses to plastic lenses—they weigh less and don't fog or steam up as much as glass.

The chief disadvantage is that the surfaces are not quite as hard as glass and, therefore, susceptible to scratching. With sensible care, it is a relatively trivial problem although some older patients seem to harbor a distinct phobia about it. To reduce the chances of random scratching, many manufacturers produce plastic lenses with a special surface hardening treatment. A further option is to layer a thin film of quartz onto the surfaces to afford reasonable scratch protection.

Another drawback to regular plastic lenses is that they are somewhat thicker than glass for a comparable prescription. This disadvantage is rapidly disappearing with the advent of high-index plastic materials which are both thin and light weight.

Thin Lenses

High-index means that more prescription power can be generated in less space, i.e., thinner. High-index glass has been available for a long time, but the development of high-index plastic materials has fundamentally changed the "look" of high prescription glasses. Very nearsighted or very farsighted people can now enjoy glasses which cosmetically look almost "normal". Many of these lenses also include extra ultraviolet filtering protection, scratch-resistance, and anti-reflection coatings. Even bifocal prescriptions can be fabricated into a thinner, lighter lens. Be aware, however, that converting to these lenses may require some adaptation beyond what is normally experienced with any new prescription.

What's Right For You?

Which lens material is right for you? Generally, one of the plastic varieties unless you have a special need. For instance, if you desire the photosensitive lenses that change with light conditions, those are mostly made of glass. (A plastic photochromic lens is discussed in Sunglasses & Tinted Lenses.) If you need to be concerned with high levels of infrared radiation, glass sunglasses are much more efficient in filtering out infrared than plastic sunglasses. When safety is the major concern, polycarbonate plastic is probably the best lens material in hazardous situations. It's also great for kids. To put it into perspective, it's the same material that's used for making "bulletproof" windows. Polycarbonate may also be used strictly cosmetically since it's a high-index material, although not as high as others.

With all the possible choices, it can be confusing. Make your selection after discussing your needs and options with the optometrist.

V

All About Contact Lenses

18

What Are Contact Lenses and How Do They Work?

There are two questions uppermost in the mind of anyone considering contact lenses: "Can I wear them?" and "Will it hurt?" There is also the understandable fear of deliberately putting something on the eye. The question of hurt is the easier to answer. You've had the experience of a tiny speck of dust irritating the eye and, by inference, you expect the much larger contact lens to be even more painful. But the cornea (the clear front of the eye where the contact fits) is very discriminating in its sensitivity. It is super sensitive to tiny particles touching it, but not to larger objects. You may find this hard to believe until you realize that a large object touches your cornea several thousand times a day—your eyelids. When contact are properly fitted they should not feel much different than your lids.

We don't mean to imply that you will feel nothing the first time a gas permeable hard lens is placed on your eye. There will be a decided sensation as the inside of your lids rub against the edge of the lens with each blink. (Notice that the sensation is from the lids, not the cornea.) With soft contact lenses, this rubbing sensation is virtually imperceptible and even the initial wearing is very comfortable.

Answering the first question, whether or not you can wear contacts, that hinges on the ability of the cornea to adapt to reduced oxygen and altered metabolism. This depends on your eyes, your prescription and, above all, the skill of the doctor. In short, most people with sufficient motivation can wear some type of contact lenses which are properly fitted.

In the past twenty years, specifically with the arrival of soft contact lenses on the scene, there has been a prodigious increase in their use. Millions of people wear them; millions more bought them and eventually put them away in a drawer. There are several reasons for these "failures", the predominant ones being poor and hurried fittings, which are then compounded by even worse follow-up care.

The lure of earning a easy buck draws many semi-professionals and quasi-experts into the contact lens field. There are unsparing advertisements in print, on television and in the yellow pages touting soft contact lenses. In our experience, teenagers are the most susceptible; they have the desire for the cosmetics of no glasses, but generally not the wisdom for informed decisions. Of course, the change-your-eye-color lenses play to this cosmetic craving. Regrettably for the potential wearer, the clever ad copy is usually superior to the knowledge and skill of the care providers. They can muddle through with mediocre proficiency because the soft lenses are initially comfortable and the wearer cannot judge the caliber of the fit. Be very cautious of any "sales" or "special deals" in contacts. Why? You're not buying a product like shampoo or lipstick! If the shampoo doesn't magically give your hair that "irresistible look" you simply try another brand next time. If the contact lenses injure your eye...

Keep in mind that contact lenses are an ongoing treatment for your particular sight problem, not a permanent "fix". The eyes must be examined periodically since even well fitted lenses may cause or mask subtle changes; poorly fitted lenses may provoke corneal damage. While it's true that pain will get your attention, not all problems start out with discomfort or decrease in sight. It is almost axiomatic that the doctor who conscientiously provides a good fitting will insist on regular, thorough follow-up care.

HISTORY: Most people are astounded to learn that contact lenses have been around since the 19th century. However, until the early 1950s, with the introduction of the small corneal lens, their use was uncommon and limited.

The first contact lenses were large, fit over most of the eye and were made of thin, blown glass. Can you imagine the incentive for someone to place a fragile hemisphere of glass on the eye? It was certainly not a matter of vanity. They were worn by people who could obtain good vision only with contacts— glasses couldn't help them.

In the 1940s, the development of a clear, transparent plastic which could be fashioned into contacts eliminated the use of breakable glass lenses. They were still big and bulky, covering the cornea and sclera (the white portion of the eye). The subsequent creation of a thin, small lens which rides on the cornea and is held in place by simple capillary attraction was the breakthrough which made it possible for many more people to be fitted.

BACKGROUND: The cornea is really a unique structure in many ways. Besides being transparent and selective in its response to irritants, the cornea has no direct blood supply. So it must get the oxygen and most of the nutrients needed by every living tissue directly from the air and tears. The tears must also wash away biological waste products. If anything blocks the air or compromises the tear film, the cornea's metabolism and transparency will suffer (and so will you).

The original hard lenses made of polymethyl methacrylate (PMMA) did not permit any air to pass through the material. The lens had to be designed to move slightly with each blink to create a pumping action to exchange fresh oxygen-rich tears for stale carbon dioxide laden tears. The newer rigid gas permeable (RGP) hard lenses, by mixing different polymers into the plastic material, allow some exchange of air. However, most of these mixtures are less wettable than the old PMMA which creates a whole new set of fitting problems.

The design of the lenses figures in both your comfort and the continued health of the cornea. A cross section view of the cornea under magnification reveals an aspheric (non-spherical) shape. The center peaks a bit and the edges near the white of the eye flatten out. A hard contact lens must approximate this shape, but only approximate it. Some lenses are made with an aspheric curvature for better alignment. If the lens is too tight, a seal will form causing swelling and cloudiness. If the lens is too loose it will slip around, rub and irritate the cornea and/or lids, and may easily fall out. There has to be a delicate balance between snugness and looseness which is achieved by controlling the contact's curvature, size, thickness, and edge bevels. When you realize that the average hard lens is 9 millimeters (1/3 inch) in diameter with a thickness of perhaps 2/10ths millimeter or less, that's a lot to build into a tiny piece of plastic.

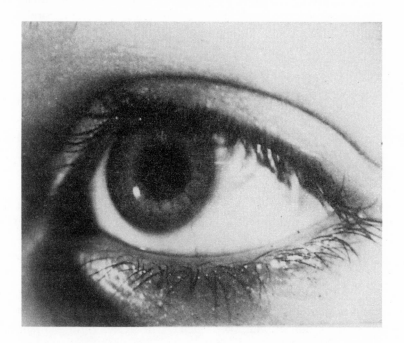

A soft contact lens in its normal position on the eye. Unlike a hard contact, the edge extends onto the white part of the eye.

A soft lens is soft because it absorbs water. Unlike the hard lens which is intended to remain within the corneal boundaries, the soft lens extends onto the white of the eye. Once on the eye it absorbs your tears, with the percentage of absorption varying from about 20% to 80% dependent on the material. The amount of oxygen and carbon dioxide diffusing through the lens depends on the percentage of water in the material and/or the thickness of the lens. The mechanism of eliminating waste products is not clear (some may be trapped) and can impact unfavorably, especially when extended-wear lenses are used.

WHY WEAR THEM? For most people, the cosmetic aspect is the underlying reason for getting contacts. Actually, there are many good reasons. Most apply to both hard and soft lenses.

1. Vision is more natural and in almost true size. With glasses objects may appear distorted in size and shape.
2. Contacts move with the eyes when you look to the sides. There is none of the distortion that you might experience with glasses.
3. Side vision is not screened by a frame.
4. When you're out in the rain or when it's snowing, the drops or flakes won't catch on the glasses.
5. Contacts won't steam up from abrupt temperature changes or perspiration.
6. If the lens correction for each eye is very different, contacts may be the only way the two eyes can work together.
7. Some people with a tendency for an eye to cross gain better eye positioning control.
8. Less frequent prescription changes are usually needed.
9. Contacts can protect an injured cornea while it heals. (Soft therapeutic)
10. As part of low vision optical systems.

There are even a few instances when contacts are the only way to get good sight: when the cornea is scarred, has an irregular shape, or in keratoconous, a disease which causes the cornea to thin and bulge. RGP lenses are generally used in these cases.

CONTACT LENS EXAM: The examination for contact lenses begins with the full regular testing of your eyes and vision, with special attention to the health of the cornea and lids. Something unusual may show up which will rule out contacts or make them a poor choice. Then specifically for contacts, the curvature of the cornea is measured. The quality and quantity of your tears is evaluated as it can have a profound affect on the choice of material and the wearing time.

DIAGNOSTIC FITTING: The examination will guide the doctor towards the proper lenses for you, but it's necessary to try several designs and materials to make the "final" choice. Usually, you'll be scheduled for a separate trial fitting to make this important determination.

19

Contact Lenses: Hard vs. Soft

In this chapter when we mention hard lenses we refer only to the gas permeable materials (RGP). The old PMMA lenses are outdated and hardly ever used anymore.

BASIC CONCEPTS: A soft lens is one which absorbs water; a hard lens does not. When a soft lens is allowed to dry it will become inflexible and brittle; a hard lens remains essentially the same either wet or dry. In fact, keeping the surfaces of RGP lenses wet on your eye is a major concern. (Manufacturers try all kinds of gambits to make their lenses wettable. Some add certain ingredients, some give the surfaces special treatments, etc.) There are many, many dozens of soft lenses and several dozen hard lenses being manufactured. It can become quite bewildering for the doctor to know the characteristics of each. Manufacturers don't exactly help by continually devising "new and improved" material combinations. How new and improved is debatable, but they do have new names.

Of much more serious concern than merely a new "catchy" name is the increased number of extended-wear, disposable lenses and daily-wear, throwaway lenses being marketed. For most people, they are an expensive, possibly dangerous, certainly a foolish, choice. Are there any benefits derived from the throwaways besides to the manufacturer and sellers? Ostensibly, by disposing of them at regular intervals, the chance of the lenses becoming soiled and contaminated is reduced. You can't dispute that argument which does, indeed, makes it beneficial for some patients. We'll elaborate on it in Chapter 21. In desperation to sell the millions of lenses that can be manufactured, companies have come up with weekly lenses, biweekly lenses, monthly lenses, three-month lenses, etc. What's next? Lenses for any month with an R in it or months with 31 days (special lenses for February)? If you believe the puffery, it would seem that "monthly" lenses don't get soiled in a week, but "weekly" ones do. How silly can it get? One potential risk comes into play when people push the wear past the intended time span, once they realize how much money they are shelling out. With the bulk of these likely being sold to teenagers, traditionally not the most meticulous age group, problems will eventually ensue.

Let's sketch a scene: Lucie, 19, has now worn her 7-day lenses for 3 weeks when she notices some irritation. "Oh, well," she decides, "I got my money's worth. Guess it's time to replace it." Since these throwaways are sold in multiple packs, she simply opens a fresh one and pops it in her eye. The discomfort continues for a few more days until the eye is in serious pain. A trip to the doctor reveals an ulcer penetrating the cornea. The point is, with regular contacts she would see her doctor for a replacement. Since no replacement should ever be dispensed without the eye being checked, the ulcer would have been caught in a very early, treatable stage. Of course, the same disaster could occur after three days of wear with Lucie assuming that the lens is damaged (and upset that she didn't get her 7 days out of it). You could certainly make a case that Lucie was stupid for ignoring the mild pain for a few days, but in reality that often happens.

Extended-wear lenses are in declining use because the potential for harm outweighs their mild benefit for the vast ma-

jority of people. There has been so much adverse media publicity (in fairness, not all justified) that few patients show much
interest in this option.

One final word: Both the extended-wear and disposable or
"planned replacement" lenses have their uses in limited cases
or special circumstances. Don't opt for them unless you belong
in this small group.

HARD, SOFT DIFFERENCES: If you pressed us for one
word which describes the difference between the hard and soft
lenses, it would be "comfort." The soft lens is delightfully comfortable from almost the first wearing. On the credit side for
the RGP lens is the usually crisper and clearer sight. Astigmatism (which most people have to varying degrees) is fairly easily corrected with a hard lens, but more difficult, sometimes
impossible to correct with a soft lens. (See "Soft Astigmatic
Lenses.") The reason is that the hard lens substitutes a firm,
round front surface for the out-of-round cornea. The soft lens
will merely drape and conform to the uneven shape, hardly
correcting the astigmatism. Also negatively affecting the sight
with soft lenses is that they can buckle slightly with blinking
or drying.

A further plus for the hard lens is its better durability since
it's barely affected by pollutants in the air. The soft lens absorbs water, your tears or anything else in liquid form. Sprays
and makeup will freely be absorbed. Someone working in a
beauty shop where sprays are constantly in use may soon find
the soft lenses contaminated and uncomfortable. Of course,
enough sprayed chemicals on the hard lenses and they, too,
will be uncomfortable. However, they are much easier to clean.

For active sports the soft lens works better (provided the sight
is good) because it's not likely to fall out of the eye; dust and
dirt cannot easily get under it.

The hard lens is essentially firm and unyielding so that with
each blink a slight pressure is exerted on the cornea. This might
have a positive or a negative side depending on whether it
induces unwanted corneal curvature changes or, as some doctors believe, restrains the increase of nearsightedness. The soft
lens generates virtually no pressure, adaptation time is quicker,
and you will be less sensitive to bright light.

As if to embarrass the title of this chapter, there is a contact lens which is a combination of both. The center is RGP with a "skirt" of soft material. It's supposed to have the crisp sight of a hard lens with the comfort of the soft.

TO SUMMARIZE: The final selection of the contact lenses best suited for you will depend on comfort, sight, occupation, environment, light sensitivity, and, perhaps, your ability to handle them. If you are still undecided and your doctor considers either type appropriate, we recommend that you try the soft contacts first. If acceptable vision cannot be obtained, then switch to the hard.

20

Guide to Successful Contact Lens Wear

I f we had to select only one indispensable ingredient for the successful and safe wearing of contact lenses, that component would be the doctor who provides a good fitting procedure, proper lens selection and satisfactory follow-up care. However, the patient also has a share in the responsibility by meticulously complying with instructions regarding the wearing schedule, handling, cleaning and sterilization of the lenses, as well as returning for periodic eye checkups at predetermined intervals.

You'll find that wearing contacts is a unique experience— first you'll learn to live with them; then you'll find it's vexing to live without them. The hints and tips in this chapter should make it easier for you.

Before leaving the doctor's office with your new contacts, make sure you know the following:

1. Insertion and removal procedures.
2. Cleaning and sterilization methods.

3. What to do in the event of an eye irritation.
4. The contact lens wearing schedule until the next visit.
5. How to center a displaced lens.
6. The normal symptoms you may experience during the adaptation period.
7. How to avoid problems when using cosmetics, hair spray; when swimming, showering, washing.

You won't have to commit everything to memory since you'll receive written information which you can study at home.

It is important, however, to know when you are developing a serious problem. With either the hard or soft lenses, the following symptoms are **NOT** normal:

1. Inability to keep the eyes open.
2. Pain during wear or after removal.
3. Unbearable light sensitivity.
4. Cloudy vision and/or colored rings around lights.
5. Harsh burning or severe irritation.
6. Eyes very red.

Admittedly, some of these symptoms vary only in degree from normal adaptation symptoms, but to be safe, remove the lenses and report to the doctor. Incidentally, you should obtain the doctor's home telephone number in case of an emergency.

Many of the following suggestions, hints and cautions apply to all contact lenses. But to make it easier for you, there are individual sections for soft contacts and for hard gas permeable contacts.

SOFT CONTACTS

In The Beginning

You'll experience almost complete comfort within a few minutes of wear. However, since comfort is only one concern, it's necessary to follow a scheduled wearing time for the first several days. With the normal daily-wear lenses, the schedule may begin at 4 to 8 hours. The doctor will designate the timetable for you to follow.

Get into the good habit of washing and rinsing your hands before handling the lenses. Otherwise they may become contaminated with body oils, cosmetics, etc.

Look at the lens carefully before inserting it into your eye. Make certain that there are no bits of foreign matter clinging to it. Then check to see if the lens is right side out. With some lenses it's very difficult to tell. Place the lens on your finger tip and look at it from the side. It should appear bowl shaped; edges flared outward means it's reversed. If your lenses have markings or lettering on the border it could be a good clue. Placing an inside-out lens on the eye will cause no harm, but it will generally feel uncomfortable and tend to move around with blinking.

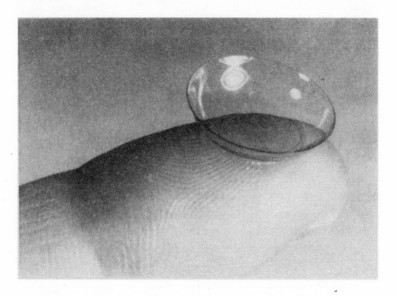

A soft contact lens in position on the finger ready for insertion.

Anyone with long fingernails must be extra careful when removing the lenses. It's quite possible to scratch the cornea and/or puncture the lens. If you're inclined to have long nails and cannot easily remove your lenses, a soft rubber removing device could be very useful.

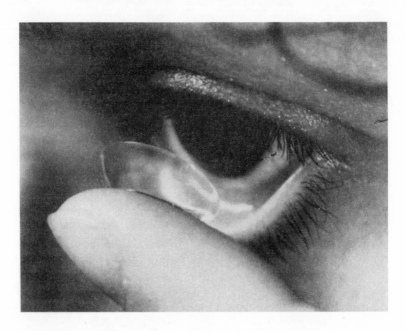

Placing a soft contact lens on the eye.

Regular Wear

Within a few days you should be comfortably wearing your contacts for most of the hours you're awake. The exact number will vary from person to person. The doctor will adjust your wearing time to both meet your needs and prevent complications.

You can modify your wear from day to day within a reasonable number of hours without any particular problem. You can even go a day or two without using the contacts.

The soft lens must absorb some water (tears) to remain comfortable. You may experience a burning/scratchy sensation if it dries for any, or any combination, of these reasons:

1. Insufficient tear supply.
2. Dry atmospheric conditions such as a heated room in winter; air conditioned room in summer.
3. Medications such as antihistamines.
4. Prolonged reading or staring which reduces the blink rate.

In may be helpful to use eye drops recommended by your doctor in these circumstances, but mostly the wetting effect is short lived. It's usually more effectual to remove, clean, wet and re-insert the lenses.

Extended Wear

Continuous wear for up to 1 week is possible with extended-wear lenses. (The extended-wear option is not highly advised for most people.) Since no one can accurately predict the cornea's physiological response to being constantly blanketed, the eyes must be monitored frequently by the doctor.

The eyes will normally dry during sleep. Therefore, a few drops of unpreserved saline at bedtime and upon arising should be beneficial.

Something In The Eye

Once soft lenses are in place, it's very improbable (though possible) for a speck of dirt or other particle to get between the lens and the cornea. The most likely time for it to happen is when you're inserting the lenses. Don't ignore any unusual sensation in the hope that it will go away. Take the lens out and rinse it thoroughly until it feels right.

Pain

Any pain must be investigated for cause. It could be a torn lens, an infection, a trapped particle, an abrasion. Lens removal is urgent which means you should always carry a storage case wherever you go. If removal stops the pain, inspect and clean the lens. If the lens doesn't appear torn and you think something might have been trapped, re-insert the lens. Persistent pain after the lens is out is a signal to leave it out and should prompt a telephone call to your doctor.

Dropped Lens

Inevitably, you will drop a lens now and again. If you insert and remove your lenses over a sink, we assume you have the forethought to stopper the sink or place a towel across it. People who forget this simple precaution may find themselves unscrewing pipes to search for a lens washed down the drain.

A dropped lens can be difficult to find because it makes no sound when it lands, may be colorless, and will cling to just about any surface. Moreover, it can spin through the air like a frisbee and land far from where you think it is. (A colored or "visibility" tinted lens should be easier to spot.) The longer you take to find it, the drier and more shriveled it will become. You may at first not even recognize it as a contact lens and wrongly think it's a piece of waste plastic. Even though you're relieved to find it, don't touch it. The lens is very brittle in this condition and can crack easily if you try to pick it up with your fingers. It should be retrieved by sliding a piece of paper under it. Then carefully place the lens in saline solution which will restore it to its pliable state. Clean and sterilize the lens before putting it into your eye. If the lens is uncomfortable, it probably was damaged and will have to be replaced.

Occasional Eyeglass Wear

There are times when you will wear your glasses—in the morning, at night, when you lose or damage a contact or when you're ill. You should have glasses with your current prescription available. Aside from the "normal" distortions you see with eyeglasses, there should be no problem switching back and forth.

Cosmetics

Generally, a woman who swaps wearing glasses for contacts is inclined to use more eye makeup. If done with care, that's perfectly all right. However, more lenses have probably been ruined by errant cosmetics than for any other reason.

Put the lenses on before applying makeup and be sure there is none on your fingers. This also applies to certain soaps which contain lotions, creams or perfumes, and leave a residue on the skin. Use a mild soap or one of the special soaps made for contact lens wearers. The eye makeup products should be water soluble; avoid getting them on the lenses. If any does get on the contacts it may irritate the eyes and contaminate the lenses.

Anything in spray form can be a disaster for soft lenses which will perfunctorily absorb the mist. If you feel the use of a spray product is necessary, close your eyes while spraying and keep them closed for at least half a minute afterwards. Better yet, move to another area or room when done. In hair salons, where sprays are freely in use, it's best not to wear soft lenses.

Difficult Wearing Times

There are circumstances when the wearing of contacts is not feasible or leads to discomfort. Smoky, hot rooms such as you might encounter during a party, can irritate the eyes. Drinking alcoholic beverages will further dry the eyes and increase the irritation. It might be helpful to step outside once in a while for a dose of fresh air.

During times of illness and when taking certain medications, it would be prudent to forgo contacts. While most women can continue to wear their lenses during pregnancy, for some it becomes bothersome.

When you resume wear, use some common sense in calculating how long to keep them in your eyes. Provided it's only been 4 or 5 days, reduce the time by about one-third the first couple of days. In the event it's been longer, follow your original schedule when you first began contact wear.

Swimming, Showering, Washing

The common denominator is the chance of too much water getting into your eyes. If you keep your head out of the water when swimming and keep you lids narrowed, you may be O.K. However, the lenses can absorb chlorinated water to irritate your eyes. The answer is to wear snug-fitting swim goggles if you prefer to use your contacts.

Keeping your eyes shut when showering or washing is generally a sufficient precaution. Obviously, avoid getting soap or shampoo in your eyes.

Careless Handling

Several factors determine the tensile strength of the lenses. Usually, a high water-content material will be more fragile. Handling a partially dry lens can create tiny cracks which lead to a torn lens. If your lenses usually feel rather dry and "sticky" upon removal, put a few drops of sterile saline into your eyes first. When cleaning, be sure the lens is thoroughly wet and watch that your fingernails don't puncture the lens.

Cleaning and Sterilization

This is a tandem which must be done regularly; one does not take the place of the other. After removing the lenses they must immediately be cleaned with the proper cleaning agent, then rinsed and sterilized. Remember, cleaning does not sterilize; sterilization does not make grime disappear.

There are two sterilization methods—chemical and heat. (Heat is not commonly used anymore.) While chemical can be used with any type of lens material, heat cannot be used with many of the high water content lenses. Follow whatever regimen was prescribed by your doctor.

Neither system is foolproof. Some people develop allergic reactions to preservatives and/or buffering agents using the chemical method. For those sensitive to the ingredients in most solutions, unpreserved saline would be an intelligent option. The thermal method won't cause any allergic reactions, but the heat may "cook" unremoved, surface-adhering protein to shorten the life span of the lens.

Soft lenses are notoriously difficult to clean when eye secretions or foreign material is absorbed. Using a weekly enzyme cleaner will minimize a buildup of protein. A heavy buildup may lead to an allergic response such as giant papillary conjunctivitis (see Chapter 43) or corneal problems. Other foreign material may simply not be removable and replacement lenses have to be obtained.

It seems that each month brings some "new" contact lens products on the drugstore shelves. The number of products is bewildering, and the temptation is to buy the one that's on sale. You might save a few nickels, but the incompatibility among products could ruin your lenses and even create eye problems. Stay with whatever has been successful and don't substitute another system without first checking with your doctor. (This brings up something that may sound trite, but many people don't know the name of what they're using—"The white bottle with the green lettering"; "The little blue bottle"; etc.)

Continuing Care

As was stated a few chapters back, contacts are an ongoing treatment for your eye condition, not a one-time reconstruction. Regular eye examinations are very important to assure safe, comfortable wear year after year.

HARD (GAS PERMEABLE) CONTACTS

In The Beginning

There should not be any pain when wearing the lenses, though you will be aware of them much of the time. The wearing schedule may begin with 2-3 hours or as much as 6-8 hours. Follow the prescribed daily increase of wearing time. You may experience periods of excessive tearing which will cause the lenses to move around more than they should. If a lens slips off the cornea onto the white part of the eye, slide it back with the instructed procedure.

There may be sensations of burning and itching. No matter how tempted, do not rub your eyes. These symptoms and other minor irritations will gradually diminish as you adapt to the lenses. If they don't, discuss it with your doctor.

Get into the good habit of washing and rinsing your hands before handling the lenses to avoid their contamination with body oils, cosmetics, etc.

Regular Wear

The number of hours you will wear the lenses every day depends on a variety of factors and could be between 8 to about 18 hours. If your maximum time is, say, 10 hours and you'd like to wear them for a late meeting or party, remove the lenses for an hour or two late in the afternoon. It should then be safe to wear them another 6 to 8 hours.

Whatever your regular wearing schedule, you should reasonably maintain it from day to day. If you normally wear them 12 hours it would be unwise to one day decide to stretch it to 18 hours as that could cause a painful abrasion.

The surfaces of the lenses must be moist to remain comfortable and see clearly. You may experience a burning/scratchy sensation if they dry for any, or any combination, of these reasons:

1. Insufficient tear supply.
2. Dry atmospheric conditions such as a heated room in winter; air conditioned room in summer.
3. Medications such as antihistamines.
4. Prolonged reading or staring which reduces the blink rate.

In may be helpful to use eye drops recommended by your doctor in these circumstances, but mostly the wetting effect is short lived. It's usually more effectual to remove, clean, wet and re-insert the lenses.

Extended Wear

Continuous wear for up to 1 week is possible with extended-wear lenses. (The extended-wear option is not advised for most people.) Since no one can accurately predict the cornea's physiological response, and the possibility of the lens "suctioning" onto the cornea during sleep, the eyes must be monitored carefully and frequently by the doctor.

Glare

There will probably be an increased sensitivity to sunlight and glare which diminishes somewhat with adaptation. Good sunglasses are almost indispensable. At night, as your pupils enlarge, you may get some sparkle or shimmering effect from the edges of the lenses. If you cannot adapt to this, the lenses may have to be changed.

Something In The Eye

It's very possible for a piece of soot or dirt to become trapped between the lens and the cornea resulting in sudden pain and tearing. A good way to remove it is to hold the upper lid firmly against the bone under the eyebrow and blink violently. If the particle resists this attempt, remove the lens, rinse it and put it back in your eye.

Pain

Any pain must be investigated for cause. It could be a damaged lens, an infection, a trapped particle, an abrasion. A sudden pain is probably SOMETHING IN THE EYE. Persistent pain after the lens is out is a signal to leave it out and should prompt a telephone call to your doctor.

Wearing the lenses much longer than your normal time could result in an abrasion of the cornea. You may be unaware of the injury until several hours after removing the lenses. Symptoms are severe pain, intolerance to light and copious tearing. Call your doctor. The only consolation is that the healing process is fairly rapid (less than 36 hours) and complications are rare. Take whatever analgesic (aspirin, acetaminophen) you normally use, and apply cold compresses over the closed lid to relieve some of the pain. A pressure bandage over the lid can keep the lid from rubbing across the injured area to a minimum. The doctor will check your eye for complications and advise you when you may resume contact lens wear.

Dropped Lens

Inevitably, you will drop a lens now and again. If you insert and remove your lenses over a sink, we assume you have the forethought to stopper the sink or place a towel across it. People who forget this simple precaution may find themselves unscrewing pipes to search for a lens washed down the drain.

Pick a dropped lens up by wetting your finger, touching it to the lens and lifting straight up. Dragging the lens will scratch it. Sometimes the lens will land dome side up and stick to the surface with suction. Pour a little water over it to float it loose and work a piece of paper under the edge. Never use a sharp object to pry it loose.

Occasional Eyeglass Wear

There are times when you will wear your glasses—in the morning, at night, when you lose or damage a contact or when you're ill. You should have glasses with your current prescription available. After removing the contacts and putting your glasses on, you may notice your sight is blurred for a short time. If this "spectacle" blur persists for more than about 15 minutes, report it to your doctor.

Cosmetics

Generally, a woman who swaps wearing glasses for contacts is inclined to use more eye makeup. If done with care, that's perfectly all right.

Put the lenses on before applying makeup and be sure there is none on your fingers. This also applies to certain soaps which contain lotions, creams or perfumes, and leave a residue on the skin. Use a mild soap or one of the special soaps made for contact lens wearers. The eye makeup should be water soluble products, and avoid getting them on the lenses. If any does get on the lenses it may irritate the eye and contaminate the lens.

Anything in spray form can accumulate on the lens surfaces making them less wettable. Close your eyes when using sprays and keep them closed for about half a minute. If your lenses do become coated, they may require resurfacing.

Difficult Wearing Times

There are circumstances when the wearing of contacts is not feasible or leads to discomfort. Smoky, hot rooms such as you might encounter during a party, can irritate the eyes. Drinking alcoholic beverages will further dry the eyes and increase the irritation. It might be helpful to step outside once in a while for a dose of fresh air.

During times of illness and when taking certain medications, it would be prudent to forgo contacts. While most women can continue to wear their lenses during pregnancy, for some it becomes bothersome.

When you resume wear, use some common sense in calculating how long to keep them in your eyes. Provided it's only been 4 or 5 days, reduce the time by about one-half the first day, then gradually build to regular time. In the event it's been longer, follow your beginning, original schedule.

Swimming, Showering, Washing

The common denominator is the chance of too much water getting into your eyes. If you keep your head out of the water when swimming and keep you lids narrowed, you may be O.K., but the lenses can float out of the eye. The answer is to wear snug-fitting swim goggles if you prefer to use your contacts.

Keeping your eyes shut when showering or washing is generally a sufficient precaution. Obviously, avoid getting soap or shampoo in your eyes.

Careless Handling

The penalty is cracked, chipped and scratched lenses. Generally, the more gas permeable the material, the easier it is to become warped, cracked and scratched. When enough scratches accumulate the surfaces will not wet properly. The dry spots cause hazy vision and some discomfort. If the scratches are not too deep, most hard lenses can be resurfaced to restore the smooth finish. Some materials cannot be resurfaced.

Cleaning and Sterilization

Immediately upon removal, clean the lenses with the prescribed cleaner, rinse and place in the soaking/sterilizing solution. The gas permeable lenses have a great affinity for attracting and retaining eye secretions. Regular weekly or bi-weekly enzyme treatment is recommended.

Continuing Care

As was stated a few chapters back, contacts are an ongoing treatment for your eye condition, not a one-time reconstruction. Regular eye examinations (preferably every six months) are very important to assure safe, comfortable ongoing wear. You should understand that after wearing hard lenses for many years, the cornea becomes less sensitive to pain; a serious condition might develop long before you're aware of it.

21

Special Lenses

Small and moderate amounts of astigmatism generally cause no sight problems with hard lenses, but may with regular soft lenses. The toric soft lens is meant to overcome this problem. However, the fitting can be tedious and difficult. The lens must be designed to remain in a predictable, stable position on the cornea. There are a only a couple of ways to do this—making part of the lens thicker and/or heavier or by making the bottom edge straight to rest on the lower lid.

Sometimes the drag of the lid when blinking or looking to the side can pull the lens off its intended position and blur the sight. Blinking can also cause flexing of the soft lens which results in an annoying variability in vision. Torics work well for some people though different designs may have to be attempted before a satisfactory one is found.

Bifocal Contacts

Hard PMMA contacts in bifocal form became available in the early 60s, although they never achieved great popularity. It's no wonder since they were troublesome to fit, required a long adaptation period, and could be unpredictable in their action. Currently, of course, the hard contact bifocals are made with gas permeable materials in several design strategies.

The soft contact bifocals have comfort going for them, but often leaves much to be desired in their ability to correct distance and/or near vision. Four types are available:

1. Reading portion at the bottom similar to bifocal glasses.
2. Central zone for distance with a gradual change in power towards the edge of the lens to provide intermediate and near sight.
3. Central zone for distance surrounded by a zone for near or vice versa.
4. Concentric grooves are formed into the lens surface to create a far and near image.

The last three types give the patient the distinct advantage of being able to read in any position rather than only in the downward gaze. However, many people experience annoying "ghost" images which are often worse at night. The bifocal with the grooves also creates some color fringes and haziness which can be very disconcerting. Strictly for sight, the one with the reading portion at the bottom is probably best provided the lens remains properly positioned.

There is no such thing as a "perfect" bifocal contact lens, whether hard or soft material, just as there are no "perfect" bifocal glasses. They all have some advantages and disadvantages which really cannot be evaluated without trying them on your eyes. If you are willing to make certain compromises, you have about a 65% chance for success.

To avoid the entire hassle of fitting unpredictable bifocal contacts or to overcome their limitations, some doctors utilize a "monovision" strategy. This means that one wears a contact for distance seeing in one eye while the other eye is fitted with a contact for near seeing. Despite some obvious loss in binocular sight and depth perception, many people adapt to this arrangement surprisingly well.

Therapeutic (Bandage) Contact Lens

This is used for the treatment and rehabilitation of certain eye diseases and disorders. Its purpose is to relieve pain, promote healing, maintain moisture and as a reservoir for continuous release of medication.

The conditions for which these lenses are used:

1.   Chemical and thermal burns.
2.   Postoperatively, i.e., corneal transplant.
3.   Corneal erosions and abrasions.
4.   Diseases of the cornea.
5.   Severe dry eyes.
6.   Deformed and defective cornea and/or iris.

These lenses are worn for extended periods of time, monitored carefully by the doctor and replaced when required.

Artificial Iris and Pupil Lens

Custom opaque colored lenses can be designed to cover a disfigured eye due to injury or disease. If the eye is capable of sight an artificial iris lens (creating a substitute pupil) (a) keeps excess light from entering; (b) reduces distortions causes by corneal scarring and (c) matches the iris color of the other eye. Improvement in sight will usually result.

If the eye is blind and is cosmetically detracting, an artificial pupil and iris can make it look similar to the other eye.

VI

Children's Vision

22

The Developing Visual System – How it Matures

The full story on how the visual system develops is unclear and incomplete. You obviously can't ask the newborn baby what and how it sees and expect a cogent answer. Experiments are difficult to devise and carry out. Nevertheless, during the last few decades great strides have been made in furthering our understanding.

It should not be surprising that the central area of the retina (light sensitive layer on the inside back of the eye) and its fovea (locus of keenest sight) continue to develop after birth until about age 4 or 5. The most significant changes occur during the first year of life, especially the first months. Thus, visual acuity and ability to fixate on an object are notoriously poor in infants, but rapidly improve. The improvement is dependent, in large measure, by good quality images from the environment reaching the retina. There seems to be a feedback mechanism which influences the growth and maturation of the retina.

As in other areas of human physiological development, the two parts of the controversy are: What is built into the system and what has to be learned. As it turns out, both play an important role. Let's trace a few of the basic steps.

The space world of the newborn infant is quite close, probably within a few feet. Most of the seeing is done with one eye at a time because the neural control of the ocular muscles is not in place. When the baby is a month old, you will notice that she's able to direct both eyes at the same near object. If you're a very careful observer, you many notice that these eye movements are jerky and uneven at first, but with practice they become smooth and facile. At this stage she will turn her head not only to follow moving objects, but also when changing fixation. In time she will learn to gain the same visual information by only moving the eyes.

By three months of age, with visual acuity rapidly improving, the eyes should be working as a team for seeing at all distances. Certainly by one year the teamwork should be well ingrained and neither eye should go drifting off on its own. With both eyes working together and receiving similar visual inputs, the stereopsis (3-dimension) cells in the brain will be activated.

Once fully activated, 3-D provides a strong stimulus for the two eyes to maintain good binocular vision.

It's fairly easy for you to check whether the baby's eyes are working together. Hold a lighted candle or a penlight flashlight about thee feet away and watch the flame/light reflection on the cornea. The reflections should be centered in the black pupil at about the same position in each eye.

A crossed eye cannot be ignored. When the child is tired, should you notice that one eye seems to be turned, or worse still, if it's constantly crossed, your child needs to be examined as soon as possible. Failure of the two eyes to work together at an early age will result in abnormal development and may result in amblyopia. (See Chapters 24 and 25.)

Most of the physical growth of the eyes occurs within the first three years of life. As the eyes grow, there seems to be an ongoing kind of compensation among the cornea, lens and size of the eyeball. Appropriate maturation of this optical system will theoretically result in a perfectly focused image on the retina. More often than not, it doesn't work out quite that well.

If you're over forty and have to hold your reading at arm's length, you can envy a fourteen-year-old who can see the same print at three inches from the eyes. At that age, she has reached the maximum flexibility of the focusing system. After that it's downhill. The importance of this flexibility will become apparent in Chapter 26.

The visual system will innately mature as long as light, forms and shapes can stimulate the retina. However, all the other senses must add their input for the brain to decipher the meaning. For example, is that round 3-dimensional object coming at you hard or soft, a basketball or a balloon? Touch and feel and sound are the ways the brain initially learns the difference. It doesn't much matter if you feel the basketball with your hands or it bounces off your head—the brain records the information. Later in life, the brain can make a reasonable assumption from only visual clues. If the object floats around, is bright green with a string dangling from it, the brain makes its "best bet" guess and chooses "balloon."

Whether an object is hot or cold takes a similar route of experience. Touch must originally be integrated into the total perception. You soon learn that seeing steam rising from a bowl of soup is a clue that it's hot without having to burn your tongue. Sometimes visual clues are not available or are inadequate. Many people are burned by electric irons because there are no visual clues if it's hot or cold.

There is evidence that size scaling must also be programmed into the brain by way of touch. Hence, when the baby "gets into" everything, she's merely coding a program to judge distances by object sizes and vice versa.

As you must now realize, the infant can "see," but what she sees lacks meaning. She slowly build a meaningful world by integrating all the other senses. Not to be overlooked when we speak of senses is body movements (including crawling) and the resulting feedback. This supplies the brain with heaps of information, i.e., how far she is from an object and where that object is in relation to others. Only by physically moving from one place to another can she learn to later judge distances with glancing visual clues.

This very brief description of the developing visual system merely touches a few of the highlights to give you an inkling of the complexity involved. When everything is put together in an orderly way it spells vision, or more aptly, perception.

23

The Examination and Treatment of the Infant and Pre-Schooler

For reasons which will become even more obvious in the next few chapters, the vision and eye health problems of the infant and pre-schooler must be detected early. We strongly urge that every child be seen routinely by an optometrist beginning at 6 months of age.

Your startled reaction might be to ask how an infant can have an eye examination and tell us what he/she sees. Indirectly, that's exactly what the infant does. One of the tidiest procedures is the preferential looking technique. While sitting comfortably on mom's lap, one eye is covered and the infant is shown a series of 10x18 inch cards with stripes on one half. The "automatic" response is for the infant to gaze at the striped pattern more than the blank side. On subsequent cards, the width of the stripes is reduced until the eye can no longer resolve them from the background. This translates into how well the eyes see, i.e., visual acuity. What we're looking for is reasonable equality between the two eyes and whether the baby's sight matches the age-expected level.

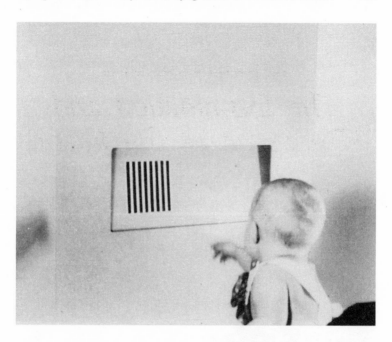

Testing the visual acuity of an infant using the preferential looking technique. The infant responds by pointing or looking at the stripes.

It's fairly easy to evaluate the eyes' centering position, ability to track moving objects and the pupil reaction to light. On the other hand, the assessment of the general health of the eyes, internal and external, is more challenging. (Infants tire quickly, fall asleep, fuss, get hungry, etc.) It may be necessary to return for a second office visit to complete the examination. Assuming everything is within a normal range during this initial appraisal, it establishes a good base-line for comparison with future examination results.

The next examination can be a year later at about the 18-month level. (Quite frankly, we prefer this age vs. the 2-year-old.) These follow-up exams are important because the child cannot tell you if something is wrong. As far as the child is concerned, it's the only way to see. Many parents assume (without really thinking about it) that the pediatrician is minding the child's vision. However, with the exception of an obvious problem which you may notice yourself, the pediatrician is not extremely knowledgeable in vision and eye care. This is not a condemnation of the pediatrician who is very busy coping with fevers, inoculations, injuries, allergies, runny noses, etc.; there is hardly time for a full vision evaluation.

As the child gets older, we can add additional and more sophisticated tests. But the objective always remains the same:

1. Are the eyes healthy?
2. Can the child smoothly move both eyes in unison?
3. Is there any tendency for the eyes to cross?
4. Is the sight maturing normally?
5. Are both eyes working together?
6. Do the eyes focus at near?
7. Is stereopsis (depth perception) present?

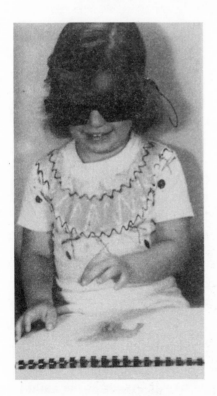

Wearing glasses with one red and one green lens, the child happily pinches an elephant seen in 3-D.

A suspected in-turning eye or out-turning eye probably brings more toddlers into the office than any other complaint. Parents present the child with the statement: "Doctor, I think Susie has a crossed eye." If the examination confirms that it actually is a crossed eye, supplemental tests will determine whether it is crossed occasionally or constantly; the amount and direction of turning. This information is fundamental in deciding on the treatment.

On the other hand, if the examination shows the eyes to be straight, the parents' observations could have been faulty, but understandably so. The bridge of most toddler's noses are flat, wide and not yet well formed; normal eye movements may give the illusion of a crossed eye. We can't overlook the possibility, however, that the child's eyes only cross when he or she is very tired. We advise the parents to continue to observe the child carefully. A history of other family members having crossed eyes is a red flag.

At 3 or 4 years of age, the sight should be almost adult-like. There are several clever ways of measuring the acuity of toddlers. One, called the BROKEN WHEEL test, disguises the letter C as "broken" automobile wheels in one car picture, while the second pictured car has full letter O wheels. With one eye patched to make the child "look like a pirate" the other eye is tested. The child merely has to say which car has the broken wheels. The presentation of the cars (and the disguised letter C) is made progressively smaller from 20/200 to 20/20. Kids love this game.

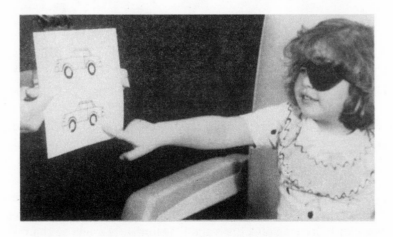

Testing the visual acuity of a toddler using the "Broken Wheel" test. The actual testing is done at 10 feet.

Though the child passes this simple acuity test, it doesn't rule out some astigmatism, nearsightedness or farsightedness. These conditions can be picked up quite readily and objectively using a retinoscope instrument and focusing a beam of light into the eye. No verbal response from the child is necessary.

In point of fact, most infants will show farsightedness and a fair amount of astigmatism, both of which we expect to fade away with normal growth.

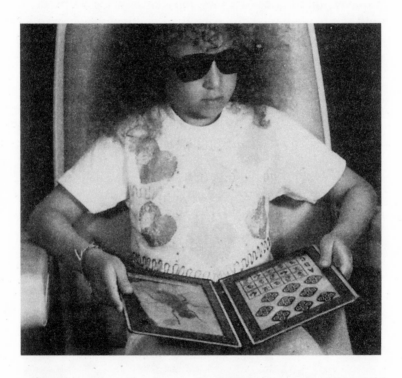

Wearing polarizing glasses, the 3-D or stereopsis of this child can be measured.

Sometime before entering preschool or kindergarten, a color vision test is given. The child with a color deficiency could be at a disadvantage if parents and teachers are unaware of the problem. Drawing pink grass and lilac tomatoes might be charming for a toddler, but the charm soon wears off if the child doesn't seem to know the correct colors.

For the vast majority of children, we find everything to be progressing normally during these early-year exams. Remember, however, that as the child grows, the eyes are growing and changing, and vision requirements become more demanding.

Normal Development

When the baby is born, the visual system already embodies built-in, hard-wired information, but you have to learn to see much the same as you have to learn to speak. Just as learning to speak is nearly impossible without getting auditory input, you cannot learn to see without light input—it's an absolute prerequisite. Bit by bit, with regular visual input, the visual system fills in the additional information needed to construct a visible world with substance, solidity, and meaning. The following takes you through the normal steps of this development, with consideration for individual variations. Note that the first two years mark the period of greatest growth of the eyes. It can be fun watching your child go through these levels.

BIRTH TO 3 MONTHS: A newborn's visual acuity ranges from about 20/400 to 20/1200 and slowly improves to approximately 20/150 to 20/600. The poor sight is because the retina is still evolving and the fovea (where the eye can see 20/20) hasn't yet matured. An adult at these levels would be in serious trouble, but for the infant, everything of interest is large and up close: mom's face and the food supply. Indeed, faces get more visual attention than anything else. True depth perception is absent. Near the end of this 3-month span, the infant will begin to exhibit simple, visually directed reaching towards objects with increasingly better results. Moving objects will also begin to attract attention.

4 TO 6 MONTHS: Visual acuity continues to improve to a reasonable 20/50 to 20/200. If both eyes are seeing about the same, stereopsis (depth perception) kicks in to nearly adult levels. Reaching for a seen object becomes proficient and tracking a moving target is fairly smooth.

7 TO 12 MONTHS: There is very little change in acuity, but other visual skills are continually getting better. The infant can

now converge the eyes as close as 3 inches and focus quite accurately.

13 TO 24 MONTHS: Visual acuity makes steady gains to the 20/30 to 20/80 range. The eyes begin to shift readily to objects of curiosity. Eye-hand coordination becomes almost flawless.

Health Problems

Any eye disease requires prompt attention. For instance, a child born with congenital cataracts must have them removed as soon as possible so light can stimulate the retina. Other conditions which can adversely affect the infant's eyes are: prematurity; diabetic mothers, taking prescribed or illicit drugs, or having AIDS, etc. Fortunately, the occurrence of possible hereditary and/or genetic disorders are not numerous. We'll briefly discuss only the few which make up the bulk of the problems encountered.

PREMATURITY/LOW BIRTH WEIGHT: Medical science has reached a stage where even premature infants of 24 weeks gestation time and weighing only 1000 grams (2.2 pounds) are surviving. These infants face very difficult impediments to growth and development. (Normal birth weight is between 2,500 and 3,800 grams, 5½ – 8½ pounds.) While prematurity and low birth weight are usually linked, the baby with a gestational age of less than 37 weeks but normal weight is still considered premature; the baby of full gestation time but less than 5½ pounds is considered in the low birth weight category.

Low birth weight other than prematurity is usually due to intrauterine growth retardation (IUGR) which, in turn, may be caused by the following factors during pregnancy: alcohol abuse (illicit drugs), malnutrition, and viral infections. Far and away the main reason for IUGR is alcohol abuse which creates a multitude of signs and symptoms under a general heading of Fetal Alcohol Syndrome. The devastating effect on the majority of these children is mental retardation because the alcohol poisons the fetus' central nervous system. Because the visual system is an integral part of the central nervous system, nearsightedness and crossed eyes are a frequent accompanying complication.

Retinopathy of Prematurity is a condition often affecting very low birth weight infants; the lower the weight, the more likely it can occur. It involves improper growth of blood vessels at the perimeter of the retina. In 90% of the cases, the situation resolves by itself while the remainder proceed to quite serious complications.

CATARACTS: Congenital cataracts are usually present at birth but may not be noticed until some future time. The cataracts can be small or large, in one or both eyes. They can remain limited or increase in size. Small, dot-like cataracts will have minimal affect on vision, but larger ones can cause blindness. Perhaps 1 in 200 infants has some form of congenital cataracts but they account for about 10% of all blindness in preschoolers.

Cataracts may also develop from eye diseases or drugs prescribed to treat systemic diseases. Long term corticosteroid use for asthma, for instance, can trigger the formation of cataracts.

Any cataract that interferes with sight must be dealt with promptly. The treatment depends on the density of the cataracts and whether one or both eyes are involved. An infant born with dense cataracts in both eyes must have them removed before 8 weeks of age to permit light stimulation of the retina.

NYSTAGMUS: This is a rapid, side to side oscillation of the eyes. It may be congenital and associated with albinism; it may be caused by some sensory deprivation earlier in life. The congenital type, while creating some sight impairment, is relatively benign. Acquired nystagmus may be caused by brain lesions and must be carefully investigated.

NASAL LACRIMAL DUCT OBSTRUCTION: About 1 in 20 babies has this condition. The drainage tube for the tears (at the inner corner of the lower lid) does not form early enough. The tears will spill onto the cheeks and an infection may follow. By 6 months of age, 80% of the obstructed ducts will open without treatment. The remaining have to be probed open.

LEUKOCORIA: The normally black pupil looks white. A number of congenital and acquired diseases can cause this appearance. The most likely are cataracts; the most serious is retinoblastoma.

RETINOBLASTOMA: This is a malignant tumor within the eye. It is a very rare condition, but life threatening. Since it's a genetic disorder, it is more likely to occur within families.

BIRTH TRAUMA: Prolonged and difficult deliveries, especially when forceps are used, may cause mechanical injuries to the eyes, eye muscles, and surrounding areas. While most traumas are mild and will clear in a few weeks, some corneal damage will cause permanent sight problems.

ACQUIRED IMMUNODEFICIENCY SYNDROME (AIDS): The route of infection can be via blood transfusion or during birth. The incidence is low but rising every year. About one-fifth of the pediatric AIDS cases have eye involvements which, sadly, may be the least of their troubles.

Mental Retardation

Many of the mentally handicapped have a high aggregate of visual problems. Since about 80% are classified as Educable Mentally Handicapped, the early detection and improvement of vision disorders for this population is extremely important to enhance whatever education is possible. (Statistics are inaccurate, but in the U.S. there may be over 4 million in this group.)

The three most common mental retardations with related vision problems are cerebral palsy, fragile X syndrome, and Down's syndrome.

Other Problems

If the health is good, what problems do we consider treating at an early age? Essentially there are four:

    1. To prevent the development of amblyopia ("lazy eye").
    2. To stop amblyopia from becoming more embedded.

3. To prevent the development and/or progression of a crossed eye.

4. To improve unacceptable blurred vision which might interfere with the normal development of good fusion (two eyes working together in harmony.)

The list is clear cut enough, but the clinical decisions often are not. How much difference between the two eyes can be tolerated? How long can the doctor withhold treatment to observe what changes may occur naturally? Is the best treatment with glasses, with an eye patch, with a combination of both? Is eye-muscle surgery indicated? Over the past few decades, some general guidelines have unfolded to aid in the decision making for various situations:

Amblyopia: This is almost always associated with a crossed eye and/or large differences in the sight of each eye. Normally, the full spectacle correction will be prescribed. A patching regimen and vision therapy can be added.

Exotropia: (One eye turns out.) The full correction with additional lens power and/or prisms to help hold the two eyes yoked together. Patching may also be needed and vision therapy when the child is old enough. Intermittent Exotropia. One eye turns out some of the time. Same treatment regimen.

Esotropia: (One eye turns in.) If the cause is considerable farsightedness and/or excessive near-focusing, the full correction is modified with either a bifocal or prisms. If needed, patching is instituted; vision therapy when the child is older. Intermittent Esotropia: One eye turns in some of the time. Same treatment regimen.

Alternating Exotropia/Esotropia. Sometimes one eye will turn, sometimes the other. Treatment is similar to one eye's turning.

The next few chapter elaborate on these issues, but in the final analysis, a large dose of professional judgement enters into the decisions.

24

Amblyopia – "Lazy Eye"

What is a "lazy" eye? Have you ever heard of a "lazy" ear or a "lazy" finger? What is unique about the visual system that permits the condition of amblyopia or "lazy" eye?

The word "amblyopia" comes from the Greek as do many medical terms; it means dull vision. In modern usage it generally refers to a particular class of dull vision with these traits: 1) there is no detectable disease, and 2) the sight is not correctable with regular lenses to better than 20/40.

Overall, there are essentially two types of amblyopia. One is caused by toxic substances such as alcohol or tobacco, the other is caused by lack of use—functional.

A detailed patient history is the best clue as to which type the person may have. The category we are concerned with here is amblyopia "ex-anopsia" (which is Latin for lack of use.) This functional variety makes up the majority seen in clinical practice.

On the face of it, not using an eye seems absurd. The eye is open so it must be seeing. Well, yes, it is seeing, but not with the high resolution of central sight. You would imagine that someone not seeing clearly with one eye would be aware of the situation and find it annoying. However, as the old classic Gershwin song declares, "It Ain't Necessarily So."

When both eyes are open, are you seeing with the right or left eye? Do you see equally well with both eyes? You might be surprised how many people have never compared the sight of their two eyes. (Patients who are being examined for the first time are often shocked when we make them aware of the difference.) It doesn't really require that much to see unequally with each eye. Minor variations anywhere along the path of light rays in the eye can be very significant. For example, an increase of the length of the eyeball of only 1 millimeter (about 1/25th of an inch) can plunge visual acuity from 20/20 to 20/400.

To deliver the best sight with true stereoscopic vision, the two eyes must work together in tight balance. What do you suppose would happen if something interferes with those balances?

Let's suppose that the brain, instead of receiving equal information input from each eye, (for reasons we'll discuss shortly), receives dissimilar information. There is a familiar adage used in computer parley called GIGO. It means garbage in, garbage out. If you feed nonsense information into a computer, nonsense answers will emerge. If you feed nonsense information into the brain, a potentially similar situation is created.

For example, if there is one tree in the road but each eye reports separately that the tree is in a different location or at a different distance, you're in a quandary. You either have to stop and use your sense of touch to establish which is the real tree, or take a 50/50 chance of bumping into that tree. The former would be tedious and painstakingly slow, the latter could be unhealthy. But the brain is much more ingenious than a computer. Since the sense of vision is so vital and because the brain is so dependent on it for information about the external world, the two conflicting inputs will not be tolerated.

Thus, the brain will gladly sacrifice the advantages of better sight and stereoscopic vision to avoid the dreadful confusion

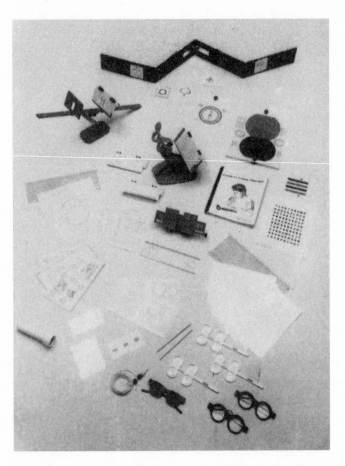

A sampling of the large variety of equipment used in vision therapy training. Many may be prescribed for training sessions at home.

of double vision. Simply put, the brain learns to ignore the input from one eye. That's not as difficult as it sounds. If, while you are reading this, you hold the palm of your hand about three inches in front of one eye, you should be able to continue reading even if you're vaguely aware of your hand. Do it long enough and the awareness of your hand tapers off. The brain is simply ignoring the input of the screened eye as you concentrate on the reading material.

Now imagine a child growing up with one eye's input being ignored for many years. The pattern would become so ingrained, that a normal binocular pattern might never be established or, if already established, might be abandoned. Even if the original cause of the problem is then removed, the brain is incapable of reestablishing binocular vision by itself. (The "binocular" brain cells physically shrink.) That's where visual therapy for amblyopia and binocularity comes in.

What would cause the two eyes to feed different information to the brain? As mentioned before, the variation in the size of each eyeball could be one reason. It's really not all that unusual when you consider that your feet or ears are probably not identical in size. Another common reason is a high degree of astigmatism or farsightedness in one eye. If the brain receives a clear image from one eye, a blurry image from the other, it will embrace the clear image and disregard the blurry one.

About two-thirds of amblyopes have an eye which is turned in or out and we'll discuss that in the next chapter. Which comes first? It can happen either from a genetic factor or the origin may be obscure.

Can the amblyopic condition be overcome? Generally it can, depending on the cause and accompanying complications, but it demands a lot of persistence. Testing must first be done to determine the exact problem. Crossed eyes and amblyopia of long duration are impeding entanglements to a successful resolution.

Treatment strategies will depend on the outcome of testing and usually follow four routes:

1. Correction of the sight problem with glasses or contact lenses.
2. Some type of concentrated stimulation (therapy) to the macula of the amblyopic eye.
3. If an eye is turned, straightening it. (Chapter 25.)
4. Building and enforcing binocular, stereoscopic vision (if possible) to keep the eyes working together.

The last three steps require diligent work by the patient. The longer the problem has existed, the more difficult the remediation. If you remember nothing else from this chapter, engrave this on your memory. An amblyopic eye doesn't cure itself. Children don't "grow out" of this disorder, they grow more severely into it. Early detection is the best way to avoid additional troubles.

25

Crossed Eyes

The expressions "cross-eyed", "squint", "cock-eyed", "tropia", and "strabismus" all refer to the same disorder—one eye does not look in the same direction as the other. In ancient times people with crossed eyes were thought to be bewitched and were treated with cruelty. We are a little more sophisticated now—we only make these people subjects of ridicule and the butt of jokes. Naturally, cross-eyed people are sensitive about their looks, but the appearance is only the visible symptom of a deeper problem.

Strabismus, the official medical term, can assume many forms. One eye can turn in (esotropia) or out (exotropia), up (hypertropia) or down (hypotropia), and even combinations such as in with up, etc. The eye may be crossed constantly or occasionally (intermittent strabismus). While the intermittent form is easier to deal with clinically, it must be evaluated and dealt with professionally.

In all cases of strabismus, one eye does the sighting while the other eye looks somewhere else. In a few people the sighting eye and turning eye will alternate roles (alternating tropia), each periodically doing the sighting.

In the majority of cases strabismus is considered to be a defect in the normal development of binocular vision in childhood. A common misconception is that crossed eyes are caused by weak muscles. While on rare occasions a paralyzed or misconnected muscle is the culprit, the muscles attached to the eyeball are very strong and the range of movements quite remarkable. Except in scarce instances, a crossed eye can move quite freely. If you cover the normally sighting eye the other eye will promptly swing into position to assume the sighting function. The real problem is that the two eyes just won't work jointly; they don't look at the same object at the same time. The reason? The brain doesn't order them to do it.

Why would the brain withhold instructions for the eyes to look at the same thing? The most likely explanation is the brain's passion to avoid double vision. Double vision can be the sequel if the individual images from each eye are fundamentally different. The brain will go to any length to avoid double vision, even if it means suppressing the central sight of one eye.

A very common type of crossed eyes that we encounter is linked to high amounts of farsightedness. This is the classic case of one eye turning inward toward the nose. The probable sequence of events runs like this: To see clearly, the farsighted eyes must use an exceptional amount of focusing power. But, since focusing (accommodation) and turning the eyes inward (convergence) work together, double vision ensues. To get out of this quandary, the brain quickly "learns" that by turning one eye inward a bit more, the image falls on a less sensitive spot on the retina which is easier to suppress. The "best" option is for the eye to turn sufficiently to place the image on the normal blind spot. Thus, only one image is seen.

Other types of crossed eyes have other causes; we don't know all the reasons. The optometrist is faced with the task of determining the nature and degree before deciding on a course of action. This requires rather extensive, specialized testing. A careful history of the patient is quite important. In some families there is a strong hereditary tendency towards crossed eyes, though relatives may exhibit different versions.

Treatment

There are roughly a dozen factors which influence the outcome for a functional cure. The term "functional cure" means that the two eyes are straight and will maintain central fixation at all distances and gaze directions, even if glasses are required. The ideal functional cure includes having normal stereopsis (depth perception) in typical, everyday seeing.

It's not always possible to reach this ideal state. Just a step down will be the individual who can maintain binocular vision "almost" all the time, but does not have good stereopsis.

Let's name just two of the factors which can sway the final results for the functional improvement—one positive, one negative. The eye which crosses occasionally is the easiest to deal with and, provided it's discovered early (before age 2), treatment results are very favorable—better than 60%. At this early stage, unfortunately, parents will often ignore the condition and hope it will go away. Of course, It hardly ever does, and valuable treatment time is lost. On the negative side, deep-seated amblyopia will reduce the odds.

The actual treatment procedures can be quite involved and it's unnecessary to explain them in detail here, but the following are the logical steps to be taken:

1. Glasses are prescribed; sometimes with bifocals for children. If necessary, we'll incorporate a prism effect into the lenses to shift the images closer together.
2. Vision therapy (orthoptics) is instituted. Because amblyopia is present most of the time, we have to first break up the suppression habit. Once there is an awareness of double vision when the eyes are not straight, the patient is trained to fuse the two images into one. As this progresses, the eyes will slowly assume a straight posture for longer periods of time.
3. Stereopsis is developed and the new vision pattern reinforced to keep the eyes from recrossing.

If these methods don't work, then surgery may be indicated. But, in the majority of cases surgery should be the last resort—not the first. If the turned eye is addressed strictly on the basis of appearance, and muscle surgery is done, the eye may "look" straight, but it probably won't "see" straight. The operation by itself (assuming good cosmetic results) will rarely restore binocular vision. More often than not the eye may cross again. A functional cure through therapy is more natural than surgical intervention. However, if it's the only option to affect a cosmetic cure, vision therapy must also be provided to help the eyes function together, and to prevent any future deterioration.

When a paralyzed muscle or a neurological abnormality is present, surgery is necessary. Usually this will have to be followed by therapy and glasses.

If your child's eyes cross, visit your family optometrist promptly. Don't wait for your child to complain. There is virtually no discomfort with a crossed eye (except the taunts of other children). Don't ignore a small degree or occasional crossing (it may increase). It may not look too displeasing cosmetically, but visually it could be just as bad as a severely turned eye. Even a small amount of squint interferes with normal three-dimensional vision and will hamper the person later in life.

26

Reading Problems Equal School Failures

This topic is quite complex and many, many aspects of it are unclear and quite controversial. Like the common cold, there are many causes and many "cures". But unlike the common cold from which you generally recover in about seven days either with or without treatment, a child with a reading problem is unlikely to recover in a week, a year, or even a lifetime. The child is trapped in a world of academic defeats, frustration, and school failures which, given time, may translate into an aversion and/or hostility toward school.

Most of us take reading for granted. We're not consciously aware of the elaborate framework which coordinates various physical and mental operations. For reading to be smooth and effortless, a sequence of steps has to be navigated which converts symbols on a page into words and, ultimately, meaning. It's a prodigious achievement which begins in the eye and ends in the brain. Accomplished readers master all the steps; poor readers stumble on one or more of the interrelated steps.

Why is the topic of reading and learning discussed in this book? Some people assume that any reading problem and hence, learning difficulties must be caused by eye/vision problems; others assume eye/vision problems are never involved. The truth lies somewhere in between and we'll try to sort out the conflicting impressions.

The Reading Process

With just a moment of thought you'll concede that reading is an artificial task imposed by our civilization. There is nothing "natural" about it, any more than there is anything "natural" about playing a piano. Just as evolution is not concerned with the ability to depress ivory keys in a specified, timed sequence, neither is evolution concerned with the ability to recognize squiggles and lines as letters and words. Quite the contrary; the visual system is inherently designed to recognize objects and movement. A live scene or picture imaged on the retina is identified by the brain straight away. (This is not meant to diminish the neural complexity of that process.) Letters and words, on the other hand, must first be decoded, which embraces several subsidiary skills: The letters have to be seen and identified; letter sounds and their combinations have to be known; finally, the sounds have to be combined into words. Once the word is decoded, comprehension takes over. Comprehension relies on knowledge of the language, grammar, word associations, and prior experience.

To underscore the importance of these conceptual differences, imagine being stranded alone on a desert island with a book written in Russian (and assuming you're not Russian.) You can clearly see each Cyrillic letter, each formed word, but regardless of how long you're at it, you will never be able to read for meaning. (Your brain can't decipher the code.) However, if you take a trip to Russia, you will easily recognize a tree or a house or the color blue despite the fact that you don't know their Russian words.

(Of course, this begs the question of how you learn to recognize visual images in the first place. That topic is sketched out in Part 1.)

There is a flood of research probing into the mysteries of the reading process, but there are so many variables that complete theories are slow in coming. (Reading researchers find themselves in the same boat as physicists probing the atom—it seems that every time a system is investigated it turns out to have several subsystems.) An appealing theoretical model presumes two independent decoding tracks (programs, in computer language) for reading information to get into the brain's "meaning" center: one for word processing and one for letter processing. The word-processing route is slightly quicker; it's on a faster track. If the word is known and frequently encountered, it will be identified *in toto* by this system. Difficult or rarely encountered words will be processed by the slightly slower letter-module.

To illustrate: The sentence, *The boy was eating an ice cream cone*, is essentially whole-word processing. The words are simple and cone is one of a few anticipated and expected nouns. (You might also anticipate sundae or bar.) Changing the sentence to *The boy was eating an ice cream pyramidal*, slows things down as you have to look at almost each letter of the last word, a letter-unit decoding exercise.

Obviously, reading is a melding of both techniques. When children first learn to read it's mostly a letter-unit process—learning the sounds and sound combinations. With experience and continual exposure to the same words their recognition becomes "automatic." As time goes by, good readers rely more and more on automatic word recognition, but new words or difficult words require letter-unit processing.

The Eyes in Reading

You might think that studying one of the basic ingredients for reading, how the eyes move along the line of print (obviously the material has to be seen) would be fairly easy. True, the physical observation part is fairly easy with computerized eye-tracking equipment but the interpretation is not.

You may be surprised to learn that when reading, the eyes do not glide along in a smooth trajectory as they would in watching a bird in steady flight. Instead, the eyes make discrete jumps, known as saccades (French for a jerking move), along the line of print, pausing on virtually each word but often skipping generic short words (a, it, the, etc.). Here's another surprise—you are effectively "blind" during the fraction-of-a-second saccade just as you are during a blink. Seeing takes place only during the pauses.

Where do the lines of sight touch down on each word? The optimum spot seems to be just right of center. Some very long words may have to be taken in sections. For example, the German language is rife with very long words which are simpler words strung together: Geisteswissenschaften or Überschallgeschwindigkeit. How long do the eyes linger at each spot? The average is about 1/4th of a second which is apparently the "decoding" time. What programs the eyes to the next landing site? How often do the eyes jump back to a previous word that may have been missed or inadequately decoded? What is the ideal time duration of gaze? Does the entire word have to be seen? Do the lines of sight of both eyes have to touch down at the exact spot? The questions go on and on.

The "seeing the print" portion—without it nothing happens—is in itself quite complicated. It all originates in the eyes with the images received on the retinas. The images seen by each eye should be clear (are certain dyslexics excluded?), undistorted, and should match closely in size and shape. When necessary, glasses or contact lenses may have to be worn to achieve this objective.

Inasmuch as reading is done within arm's reach, the eyes must focus to that distance. If the page is at fourteen inches, the focus should not be vaguely at twelve or sixteen inches. Normally, children have a very abundant and flexible focusing system and need to use only a fraction of their capability. The unused portion can be considered as held in "reserve". However, to bolster and sustain both eyes working together, certain children seem to be burdened with using most of their reserve to keep the print in focus. The difference can be likened to taking a leisurely stroll as opposed to chasing after a departing train. Such children will fatigue after a short reading time.

Let's suppose that the focusing is good. By itself, that's just not enough. The eyes must carry out accurate saccades in a rhythmic left to right sequence. (For Arabic or Hebrew, right to left.) At the end of a line, the eyes have to jump to the beginning of the next line down. Moreover, both eyes should look at the same spot at the same time which involves accurate signals from the brain to the twelve muscles which position the eyes.

Superimposed with the back and forth movement the eyes must also converge—turn inward—to look at the print else the person will see double. As with focusing, if convergence has to be sustained at full capacity, fatigue will readily set in.

OK, let's assume there is a clear image of the letters centered evenly in both eyes. What happens next? Two visual subsystems are involved for detecting the letters and words—transient and sustained. The explanation is much too lengthy and complicated to entertain here except to bring out that the precisely timed interaction of the two systems is a key factor that makes normal, good reading possible. After the words and/or letters are detected, one of the two processing programs discussed previously (letter vs. whole word) takes over.

Poor Readers

Here is where we tread on soft, shifting ground. Labeling a child as a poor reader means different things to different people. Is the youngster a slow learner, a reading underachiever, reading disabled, learning disabled, have an attention deficit, or the neurological description—dyslexic?

Let's attach some definitions, even if not everyone agrees, so you'll at least have a reference point. Assuming an average I.Q., a child is expected to read at his/her grade level as determined with standardized tests. Reading below this level profiles and tags the child a poor reader. But the tag does nothing to illuminate the underlying problem.

Generally speaking, we can divide poor readers into two groups. One is the slow learner whose I.Q. is below average. The intellectual ability just isn't there, and reading is one of the many subjects below average. This borders on learning disability. The second division is the underachiever in reading whose reading performance falls short of what is expected from the I.Q. scores. It's the latter group which draws much attention from educators and/or parents.

This underachiever group can be further divided. The student with a reading difficulty or problem is the one with a surmised identifiable cause. The cause can be from emotional difficulties, poor instructions, social disadvantages, vision and hearing disturbances, and very often a combination of two or more of these.

The remaining subdivision is known variously as reading disability, specific reading disability, dyslexia, and by several other names. The common link is the presumption that the cause is a central nervous system dysfunction, best known by the designation, dyslexia. Here we find ourselves in another quagmire trying to accurately explain dyslexia which, to the general public, has become an almost generic term for any learning disability.

However, learning disability itself was defined by the Federal Government when Congress passed the Education For All Children Act, Public Law 94-142 in 1975. The definition was later revised and now reads: Learning Disabilities is a generic term that refers to a heterogeneous group of disorders manifested by significant difficulties in the acquisition and use of listening, speaking, writing, reasoning, or mathematical abilities. These disorders are intrinsic to the individual and presumed to be due to a central nervous system dysfunction. Even though a learning disability may occur concomitantly with other handicapping conditions or environmental influences, it is not the direct result of those conditions or influences.

Sorry if that doesn't clear things up too much. However, since the law went into affect, school districts have been forced to "do something" with this group of children and special education is a growing industry and an increasingly large budget item. (It has also spurred research.)

Dyslexia

As long as we're working with definitions, let's start with the "official" description by the World Confederation of Neurology: A disorder manifested by difficulty in learning to read despite conventional instruction, adequate intelligence, and adequate sociocultural opportunity. It is dependent upon fundamental cognitive disabilities which are frequently constitutional in origin. That's painting it with a broad enough brush to cover nearly everything.

Part of the general confusion is because dyslexia is not a single entity, but several. Identifying which particular one affects a student is fundamental (but too often vague) in establishing the therapy and improvement potential. For our purposes, we can subdivide dyslexia into three categories:

1. Dysphonesia, the largest group, is an "auditory" type making it difficult for the child to analyze a word by its sound. Words are recognized by sight, but deciphering unfamiliar words is laborious.

2. Dyseidesia is the "visual" stage of poor sight recognition of words and poor visual memory. There is strong evidence that this category is genetic in origin and affects four times as many boys as girls. It could account for the clinical observation that more boys have near-intransigent reading problems.

3. Dysnemkinesia is a "motor" dysfunction principally affecting handwriting with reversals of letters and numbers. This, in isolation, may not directly affect reading, but drives teachers and parents to distraction.

There is nothing to keep these three from overlapping; to preclude a child from having more than one dyslexic condition. There is also the possibility that dyslexic states "ebb and flow" from time to time.

Screening tests are available for detecting dyslexics. If the child fails the screening, a full diagnostic test is given to determine which type of dyslexia (or combination) is involved.

A psychological comment is in order at this juncture. While being identified as a dyslexic would appear to be a verdict of doom for the child, it is tolerable and acceptable for the parents because it allays any guilt feelings they may have about the "nurture" of the child. After all, a neurological problem is "nature", "in the genes" and beyond their power to control. One is left to wonder how many kids are labeled as dyslexic without a solid diagnosis just to appease anxious parents.

Signs & Symptoms

It's easy to create a checklist of children (or adults) with reading/learning problems, regardless of the exact nature of the problem. This list is not in any order of frequency and mentions only the most conspicuous presentations.

- Holds the book very close.
- Squints a lot.
- Loses place while reading.
- Covers or closes one eye when reading.

- Turns the head to block out one eye.
- Headaches during or after reading.
- Moves head back and forth.
- Rubs eyes a lot.
- Has difficulty remembering, identifying and reproducing basic geometric forms.
- Fatigues easily.
- Skips words when reading.
- Reverses letters or words after about age 5.
- Avoids reading and homework.
- Is below expected reading level.
- Has very poor handwriting; words are crowded.

The last five items are the ones to catch the notice of the parents. Most of the other symptoms are easily overlooked unless spotted by a perceptive teacher.

Most likely the child will exhibit several of these indicators posing the challenge of which came first and which are secondary. Of course, the reasons for the first 7 or 8 on the list should have been discovered with a thorough, professional eye examination long before this sorry point is reached. It's another strong argument (which can't be repeated often enough) for early (before age 2) and subsequent regular child vision exams.

Remedies & Remediations

If you look at the chart POOR/SLOW READERS at the end of the chapter, it should be apparent that some of the solutions are educational, some are psychological, some are political, some are optometric, and several are composites. It should also be apparent that the causes do not have equal weight or equal relevance. For instance, poor instruction might be valid in certain regions and isolated cases, but it probably isn't a major factor across the board. Furthermore, many components interact and the chart could easily have had a maze of connecting arrows. Example: a slow learner with a low I.Q. will be additionally burdened if a vision difficulty and/or emotional problem exists.

Psychological and political remedies are outside our scope. We will briefly describe some of the educational approaches, but spend the most time on the visual and optometric aspect.

One critical point needs to be made very early—optometrists do not teach reading. If there is a visual defect which interferes with the reading process, that obstacle will be removed, if possible, so that qualified educators can teach reading.

By now we should have made it sufficiently plain that the causes are hardly ever clean-cut, but for the sake of some semblance of order we'll divide the remedies by categories.

1. Problem or Difficulty. Vision Disorder.

Clinically, this is probably the most usual history we come across in the optometric office: the child has a normal or above-average I.Q. but is reading far below the grade level. Vision testing will reveal a binocular problem such as a focusing irregularity or inconsistent teamwork between the two eyes (oftentimes both factors are involved) which creates interference or "noise" in the very initial detection stage. At its worst, this will confuse the identification of word images; at best, it can cause discomfort after a short reading time—15 or 20 minutes. These binocular symmetry problems are not to be confused with a sight problem—mostly these kids have good distance sight.

Regard this a forewarning: The vision examination has to thoroughly cover all the facets of binocular vision (see Chapter 12), plus selected special tests. (These have to be carried out without dilation.) A cursory exam based on distant 20/20 sight is almost a waste of time.

As a matter of fact, there are many adults who have floundered through school somewhere between the "worst" and "best" scenarios. They just never tumbled to the idea that reading shouldn't be a chore—that it could be enjoyable. We've examined countless people in their 20s and 30s who present for a "routine" checkup without any specific complaint. The examination results expose a binocular vision problem and, upon questioning, the patients will acknowledge shunning reading whenever possible. They vividly recall being called "lazy" and "slow" in tackling their homework, or more likely, they tried to avoid doing homework. Avoidance is a normal animal response to discomfort. You are not going to be cheerful walking long distances with a pebble in your shoe. Neither are you going to be a happy reader with vision discomfort, though it's not as obvious as a pebble. (The lucky individuals are those we can pinpoint in grade school, before their scholastic potentials are in shambles.)

The treatment will involve glasses and/or vision training, the main objective is to remove the stumbling block to the comfortable, effortless detection of the printed material. Although the treatment plan can be summed up in one sentence, the actual remediation is a slow, often painstaking effort.

If vision training (therapy) is instituted it can take two different paths. The "traditional" training will concentrate on building and expanding the binocular skills mentioned above. It's usually achieved within the relatively short time span of a few months. Afterwards, special-use glasses may be necessary to maintain the improvements.

The second path is taken by developmental optometrists. Their core belief is that most vision disorders and learning problems are a result of poorly mastered development skills (visual-perceptual, eye-hand coordination, etc.) during the infant and toddler years. Their solution is to rectify the patterns via suitable therapy.

Which way is better? It probably depends on the severity of the deficiency. The traditional approach will work quite well with modest problems; entrenched difficulties may require the extensive program. It's one of the unresolved controversies in this topic.

As for the child, even after the vision disorder is corrected or at least skirted, the student must receive reading instruction in an attempt to catch up with his/her peers. The key is not to wait until the reading has slipped two to three years below grade level before seeking help. That may be too much of a mountain to climb.

2. Dyslexia.

Dysphonesia is the auditory, or more precisely, the auditory-linguistic type of dyslexia and the largest subgroup. Since this person finds the sounds of letter combinations difficult to decode, the treatment approach is to concentrate on sight recognition of whole words. At least this gets the child reading. Later on, teaching phonetics can be attempted. The strategy usually is quite effective in improving reading skills.

Dyseidesia is just the opposite; whole words are difficult to recognize. Reading is very deliberate and tedious because so many words have to be decoded letter by letter, sound by sound. The latest research indicates that dyseidesia is a dominant genetic trait and not curable. Nevertheless, it's possible to help the individual to work around the problem with indirect educational therapy. There are a number of remedial reading concepts, each with its adherents. The methods all rely on a variety of multi-sensory techniques of intensive instructions.

Developmental optometrists, mentioned previously, tackle the problem with visual-perceptual-motor and gross-motor training. Successfully completing the therapy program will, ostensibly, establish skills needed for reading.

What works best? Every method works for some; no method works for all. This is small solace for parents, but not all issues have open-and-shut answers. You should also realize, however, that being a dyslexic of any type does not crowd out the strong possibility that there could also be a binocular vision problem. The dyslexic hardly needs the additional millstone of a sight-detection fault. A comprehensive vision exam is a prerequisite before remedial teachers take over.

Dysnemkenesia shows up as letter reversals and scraggly handwriting. Learning good directionality (left/right) and other motor skills is quite effective in improving this disorder. Poor directionality may also effect reading, but plays a minuscule role. Developmental optometrists concentrate heavily on directionality training and can nicely manage this problem.

Other Remedies

It is difficult to predict what future research will uncover which may lead to other remedies. A curious result of some limited investigation is that "reading disabled" individuals improve their reading performance when the print is a little blurred! (Blurring the print for good readers decidedly hampers their efficiency.) The explanation could lie in the timed interaction of the sustained and transient systems mentioned briefly before. By blurring the print, the reasoning goes, the systems are timed more favorably. The timing effect could also be the explanation for the employment of colored filters and overlays which draw anecdotal raves from users and providers. Does that mean optometrists should deliberately blur the near vision of poor readers? This seems to go against the grain of providing clear images for both eyes. Time and years of research may tell.

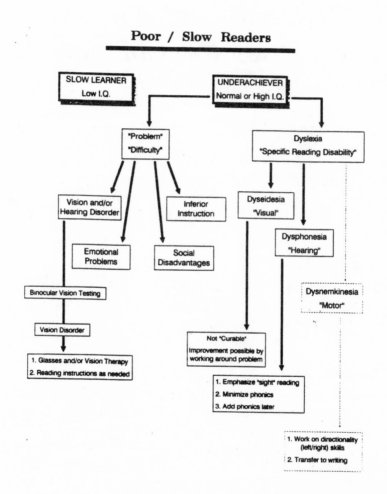

27

Bifocals and Contact Lenses for Children

You know that grandma and grandpa wear bifocals, and if you have reached the age when reading is difficult, you may also be wearing them. But have you ever heard of kids wearing bifocals? Bifocals are usually associated with older people whose ability to focus their vision on near objects such as in reading and sewing, gradually decreases. The reason, as you may recall from an earlier chapter, is that over the passing years, the lens within the eye loses its elasticity. You may also recall from an earlier chapter that children between the ages of ten and fifteen have very generous and flexible focusing ability. Why then would it be necessary to prescribe bifocals for kids?

There are four possible reasons:

1. When the ability to focus with both eyes is poor.
2. To prevent the possible crossing of an eye.
3. As a possible therapeutic step to slow down the increase of nearsightedness.

4. When focusing is weakened because of disease or medication, or entirely absent.

First, let's consider the child who has difficulty reading because of poor focusing ability with the two eyes together. This child may complain that print blurs or doubles; may get headaches or eyestrain after reading longer than a few minutes. Or, the parents may seek consultation because the child is doing poorly in school and dislikes reading.

The examining optometrist will find test results which are fairly typical in these cases. With each eye independently, the focusing ability will be normal; when both eyes are tested together, the focusing ability is much reduced. A seeming contradiction, but it's not at all unusual. The easiest way to solve this is with reading glasses for close work. However, reading glasses will make the chalkboard blurry and the glasses must be removed to see far away. To avoid the nuisance of constantly putting the glasses on and taking them off, bifocals may be prescribed.

This works quite well, but it's not necessarily a permanent solution. Visual therapy should be employed to restore the natural focusing capability. If this is accomplished the bifocals will no longer be needed.

Another need for bifocals is when one eye is crossed inward either constantly or occasionally. The bifocals make it possible to keep the eyes straight and working together. We might also prescribe bifocals when the examination reveals that one eye is at risk to cross.

Let's now consider the nearsighted child who needs frequent changes to ever stronger glasses. This child is usually an excellent reader and enjoys school. As the nearsightedness progresses the glasses get ever thicker. There is a body of opinion which feels that nearsightedness is caused by cramping of the focusing muscles during reading. It is reasoned that lessening the focusing effort with bifocals can slow the progression. (See Chapter 29, Control of Nearsightedness.)

Prescribing bifocals for kids to counterbalance disease or medication use is quite rare. Disease may cause a paralysis of the focusing muscles; the internal lens may be missing due to a birth defect or cataract removal. Some medications cause reading to blur as a side effect. Bifocals are helpful if the medication must be taken for an extended period.

Bifocals are not just for old folks, but of definite value in other cases. As long as there is parental encouragement, kids will adapt quite readily.

Contacts for Children

Once considered an unusual practice, fitting very young children for contact lenses is becoming more commonplace. With the wide variety of contact lens materials available and a young child's quick adaptation to new things, age is no detriment to contact lens wear if necessary.

Extraordinary as it may sound, infants at times need contacts. Why? These are some of the reasons: After cataract surgery, if there are large differences in the correction of each eye, extreme nearsightedness, a crossed eye, or congenital defects of the cornea and/or iris. These same conditions can exist for the pre-school or grade school child, as well.

For comfort, better stability and safety, soft lenses are by far the lenses of choice. They are essentially the same as contacts for adults except they are made smaller. In rare instances when sight cannot be improved with a soft lens, fitting a hard, gas permeable lens may be attempted.

If contacts are required for your young child's visual welfare, it will demand your calm support and supreme patience. You will probably have to insert and remove the lenses, maintain their hygiene, and watch carefully for any signs of problems.

Naturally, periodic examinations are essential for preserving the good health and vision of the growing child. The contact lenses will have to be changed as the eyes grow and the visual requirements change.

VII

Visual Therapy

28

What Is Visual Therapy?
When Is It Indicated?

Visual therapy refers to any type of active treatment procedure intended to correct shortcomings within the visual system. (It's also known as orthoptics, vision training, eye exercises.) The shortcomings in question can produce such things as a conspicuous crossed eye, an unsuspected amblyopic ("lazy") eye, reading difficulties, poor eye coordination, muted depth perception, etc. The active treatment may only involve spectacles worn as directed; or it may require a combination of prism lenses, bifocals, eye patching, light stimulation, and eye exercises.

We use the word "exercise" for lack of a better one, but don't think of it as calisthenics. The eyes are never at rest and always moving, so the twelve steering muscles get lots of physical exercise. Even during sleep there is a period of REM—rapid eye movements. Instead of thinking "exercising the muscles", think of visual therapy as a way to alter and modify the nerve impulse network within the brain's control center which govern eye movements. In computer language, think of it as modifying or rewriting a software program.

(In rare cases when eye movement is restricted by a paralyzed or "trapped" muscle, simple physical effort won't restore mobility.)

To make the important distinction clear, we'll use the analogy of learning to type. When you practice you do more than just exercise your fingers. What you're actually doing is teaching the brain to send an appropriately timed signal to the correct finger to depress a selected key. At first it's necessary to concentrate on each finger, but as you become proficient, typing becomes "automatic." When you make a typing mistake it's caused by the brain sending the wrong or out-of-sequence signal, not because your finger is weak.

Unlike a typing error, the brain's visual system can send "wrong" signals on purpose, not accidentally, to avoid a tug-of-war among the subsystems of clear sight, focusing and eye movement. The result is some degree of departure from normal vision; the most flagrant departure is, of course, amblyopia with a crossed eye.

Despite the fact that a crossed eye is cosmetically objectionable and deprives the person of normal depth perception and maximum sight, as far as the brain is concerned it's an elegant solution for avoiding double vision. Even better, a crossed eye will not cause disturbing binocular symptoms such as headaches, fatigue, reading problems, etc. These symptoms only show up when an eye is almost crossed, when the sight from one eye is almost suppressed, when the ability to focus the two eyes together is almost adequate.

The normal, comfortable, three-dimensional vision many of us take for granted is composed of dozens of complex interwoven functions working quietly in the background. Like a finely-tuned automobile engine, we're hardly aware of it while cruising along the highway with everything humming. However, if a cylinder or two stops functioning, the engine may still operate but with a decided sputter and much reduced efficiency. When another cylinder or two becomes defunct, the engine will stop. In visual terms, a minor flaw will "merely" cause headaches or fatigue; a major flaw could lead to a crossed and/or amblyopic eye.

To give you a better appreciation of the complexity, we've

listed the essential visual acts to reach the goal of normal, binocular vision.

1. Each eye must see clearly.
2. Each eye must have free movements in all directions.
3. Each eye must see comparable images.
4. Both eyes must look at the same object.
5. The brain must fuse the separate images from the two eyes into one impression.
6. The fusion must produce stereopsis—"solid" depth perception.
7. The focusing and eye aiming systems must be in congenial balance.
8. There must be an ample ability to maintain this balance for long periods of time.

A cross-eyed child, for instance, may be performing with only the first two faculties. It will be a long and difficult road to rehabilitate that visual system to progress all the way to stage 8. However, an accountant who experiences discomfort and headaches working overtime during "tax season", may be struggling with only the last two faculties—the rehabilitation will be much easier. Other kinds of visual disorders will fall somewhere in between with varying prospects for a "cure."

Parents get quite upset over a crossed eye, and rightly so, but usually for the wrong reason. They view the crossed eye as a cosmetic problem like buck teeth. If the turned eye is addressed strictly on the basis of appearance, and muscle surgery is done, the eye may "look" straight, but it probably won't "see" straight. The operation by itself (assuming good cosmetic results) will rarely restore binocular vision. More often than not the eye may cross again. On the other hand, if the two eyes are induced to work together through visual therapy, they will point straight and see straight. (There are cases when a combination of surgery and therapy are undertaken with admirable results.)

Whether the problem is amblyopia or discomfort, the training begins at the level attained by the visual system, then gradually works up through higher levels. Success depends a great deal on the motivation of the patient and persistence during the duration of the training. Although complete success is not always possible, the patient needs to make the effort or else be resigned to remaining visually handicapped.

There are five visual subsystems which training strives to improve: (a) seeing clearly; (b) focusing at all distances; (c) moving the eyes to the object of interest; (d) combining the two images into one; (e) integrating eye movements with focusing.

Many procedures and instruments are available for each stage of the therapy. There are dozens of different instruments which do similar things, but are interchanged to keep the patient from getting too bored. We'll describe some of them in general terms. The following classification has been created for your better understanding of visual therapy. In actual practice the categories tend to overlap and several functions may be trained at the same time.

Stimulating an Eye to See

Generally, an amblyopic eye requires a much stronger corrective lens than its partner. Prescribed glasses must be worn at all times. This alone, however, is probably not enough to restore sight, so we must find some additional means to provoke the eye to see. The simplest, most traditional, and moderately effective treatment is eye patching. Covering the better eye will force the amblyopic eye into action and goad it into seeing. However, since the amblyopic eye sights with an off-center, less sensitive part of the retina, patching the good eye may sometimes reinforce the bad habit and doom the effort. To get around this obstacle, most doctors will alternate patching between the two eyes on a set schedule. Sometimes it isn't even necessary to completely patch an eye; partially blocking the view of one or both eyes can work well.

A more dynamic way to eliminate amblyopia, to stimulate the eye, is to present it with some type of intense white light, colored lights or rotating patterns. Featureless light has the advantage of being acceptable to the brain since it doesn't cause any visual conflicts and thus, avoids the need to suppress the image.

Some doctors favor a method which paralyzes the focusing of the good eye with drops of a cycloplegic agent, thus forcing the amblyopic eye into service when reading. There are pro and con arguments for this one which we won't go into since this method is not widely practiced.

Focusing

Normal focusing is an automatic reflex and cannot be trained. However, the speed and flexibility of the focusing response, and its relationship to eye convergence can be altered beneficially.

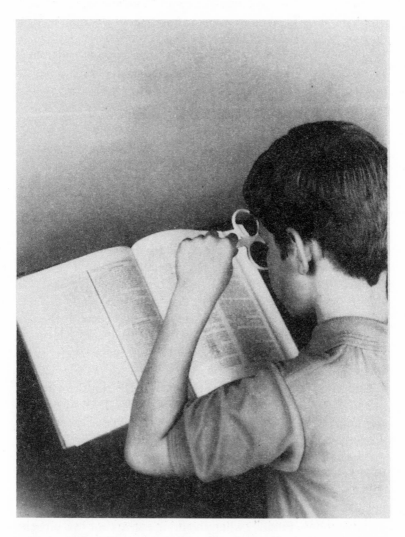

This training procedure uses lenses in a flipper holder to improve focusing flexibility when reading.

Eye Movements

There are several types of eye movements necessary for good vision. Each eye must be able to track moving objects, change fixation smoothly and accurately, and both eyes must move in unison. Since the tracking ability is dependent on a relatively clear image being seen, an amblyopic eye is usually a poor tracker. The treatment involves looking at rotating targets with, perhaps, a device for hand/eye coordination. Hand/eye coordination is used in many training procedures—it helps to reinforce the feedback. (An audible signal is substituted at times.) The eye will also be given fixation drills so that it can shift briskly from one point to another.

Fusion—Combining 2 Images into 1

It would seem that there's a contradiction in the visual system—there have to be two separate, slightly offset images available for the brain to perceive one three-dimensional object. Indeed, it's so. These closely matched images from each eye provoke specialized cells in the brain which fuse them into a sense of depth and substance. Simultaneously, the two images are "erased" to avert double vision.

In the cross-eyed child the brain ignores (suppresses) the image from the turned eye and the specialized cells are not stimulated. However, poor fusion and suppression can even exist with seemingly straight eyes. The first order of business is to eliminate the suppression and to make the brain aware of an image from each eye simultaneously.

Suppression and/or a turned eye usually develops in order to avoid seeing two objects when there is physically only one. In training, we get around this barrier with a bit of trickery. First we present large, dissimilar targets to each eye. The brain has no need to ignore either picture since they are not in conflict—they differ only minutely in color or shape or simple form. Over a period of weeks, the differences in the targets are slowly reduced—they're brought closer together, made more similar and more complex. Finally, when the brain can accept two closely matching targets, three-dimensional vision is kindled. The depth perception will be feeble, but can be strengthened with continued training.

Balancing Eye Movements with Focusing

If you hold this book about twenty inches away and slowly bring it nearer as you read, your eyes will: (a) increase focusing power to keep the print clear and (b) increase convergence to keep the print centered for each eye. (If you can relax your fusion by imaging you're looking far away, you'll see two.) A given amount of focusing is coupled with a given amount of convergence. Sometimes the coupling ratio is out of trim.

Fortunately, these linked systems have a reasonable flexibility which makes it possible, when called for, to alter the focusing/convergence relationship. This flexibility is an important factor in maintaining clear, comfortable vision, particularly at prolonged close work such as looking at a computer screen for hours on end. If necessary, to ease discomfort, the flexibility and reserve capacity can be expanded by either using a combination of prisms and lenses, and/or training (with polarized pictures, mirrors, and a score of other devices.)

Program Completion

The successful conclusion of a visual therapy program does not mean you're set for life. Like the baseball player who goes through spring training then takes batting and fielding practice before each game to retain proficiency, slumping visual skills may need refreshing from time to time. Another reason for retraining could be a change in occupation demanding different vision abilities. The good news is that retraining takes much less time and effort than the original sessions. Another approach for minimizing a slump is to wear glasses prescribed for specific seeing tasks.

29

Control of Nearsightedness

Nearsightedness, or myopia in medical jargon, has always received more attention than farsightedness. We don't have to search for the reason—myopia is quite easy to diagnose, even self-diagnose. Myopia simply means that distance sight is poor but close-up sight is good. Sooner or later the nearsighted youngster becomes aware of a deficiency; friends can read signs and recognize faces much farther away. When the child is in the classroom and has difficulty reading the chalkboard, the teacher is alerted. The eye chart hanging in physician's offices and school sight screenings will catch mostly myopes. If the nearsightedness develops in high school, the myopic teenager will fail the driver's license sight test.

Since myopia is easy to diagnose, most myopes in the population are identified. This is not so with other vision defects. (In the classroom setting, for instance, the farsighted child with a reading problem is not recognized as needing vision care.)

Because of its stubborn tendency to increase during the growing years, there is a great amount of attention given to myopia. In an attempt to avoid the steady increases, almost a century of efforts can be traced to halt, control or reverse myopia.

Overall, these efforts have been disappointing. While it's true that we have succeeded with some individuals, the percentage of myopes has been steadily increasing in the past 50 years. There seems to be little doubt that this "epidemic" is a by-product of our culture.

Scientific studies strongly suggest that myopia is directly related to the act of reading, eye focusing, illumination, head and body posture, and nutrition. The single biggest factor is probably related to reading or concentrated close work of any kind. One interesting investigation revealed that Eskimo children who historically had a low incidence of myopia, showed a remarkable increase once they were required to attend school. A current theory holds that the continuous focusing exertion at near, especially with the head downward (as leaning over a desk), causes an increase in the fluid pressure within the eye. The pressure, in time, enlarges the eyeball. Indeed, the typical myopic eye is large and out of focus for distance seeing. But, you might ask, what about the Eskimo children's poor lighting conditions during reading, or the change in their diets?

At this point, we should consider whether myopia is really a handicap. Think about the nearsighted person who is very much at ease with reading and close work such as looking at a computer monitor. Later in life, when the middle-aged farsighted person requires reading glasses, the myope is still blissfully reading without them. The major obstacle for the myope, then, is seeing clearly far away when driving, watching TV, etc. This can easily be taken care of with glasses or contact lenses. But (and this is a big but for some people), there are some psychological and prejudicial handicaps. Ever since Herman Snellen standardized the measurement of visual acuity more than a hundred years ago, the magic of 20/20 sight has made those with a lesser measurement feel inferior. The wearing of glasses was associated with "weak eyes," a silly prejudice which still exists in some quarters. On balance, the wearing of glasses or contact lenses might be a nuisance at times, but small amounts of nearsightedness is not a calamity.

We can classify myopia into four categories:
1. Simple.
2. Moderate to high.
3. Degenerative or pathological.
4. Pseudo-myopia.

1. Simple: About eight out of ten myopes fit into this group. The nearsightedness starts somewhere between the ages of seven and ten and progresses slowly for the next decade. Small increases in the strength of the prescription are needed every twelve to eighteen months, usually depending on the youngster's rate of growth. Spurts of physical growth will produce spurts in myopia. The bulk of the changes are over by the age of twenty unless the person is involved in excessive close work which may push the myopia a little higher.

2. Moderate to High: About two out of ten myopes are in this group. It starts a little earlier than simple myopia, and the changes are more frequent and greater in amount. Spurts in growth produce proportionally greater spurts in myopia and it usually levels off later in life. The higher myopia denotes a larger eyeball which causes some stretching of the paper-thin retinal layer at the inside, back of the eye. Because of this, there is a higher possibility that degenerations or detachments of the retina may occur later in life.

3. Degenerative or Pathological: This rare condition starts at birth or very early in life. The changes are rapid, large and continue into middle age. There are frequent, serious complications which can lead to sight loss.

4. Pseudo-myopia: Unlike the three previous categories, this is not a true nearsighted condition even though distance sight is poor. The muscles controlling eye focusing at near become "cramped" from excessive close work and cannot fully slacken as they should when you look far away. If this condition continues for a long time, the muscles will maintain a semi-tautness and produce a false, or pseudo-myopia. It can do such a good job of mimicking nearsightedness, that it has even been known to mask an underlying farsightedness. With appropriate and persistent testing, the doctor should be able to determine the true character.

Offsetting nearsightedness with glasses is necessary for the individual to function in our society. Unfortunately, the glasses can do nothing to stop true myopia from increasing. It will increase whether or not you wear your glasses, whether or not you eat carrots, whether or not you practice Yoga, etc.

While we tend to blame reading as the major cause of myopia, obviously not everyone who reads becomes nearsighted. There are other unknown factors. Heredity probably plays a big role—some people are just more prone than others. If we ever discover all the reasons for myopia, a true control may be possible. In the meantime, a lively debate is in process in the professional community over a number of methods which claim to prevent, halt, or reverse myopia. They are:

1. Discontinuing close work entirely.
2. Prescribing glasses with less power than testing indicated.
3. Wearing bifocal glasses.
4. Wearing contact lenses.
5. Orthokeratology.
6. Visual therapy.
7. Drug therapy.
8. Surgical procedures.

Let's examine and try to evaluate each concept. The first choice, discontinuing close work entirely or even partially, is impractical in our highly technological society. The abstinence from reading might preserve clear distant sight, but the cost would be illiteracy, a poor trade off. Besides, since we do so many things at close range, it's no guarantee for avoiding myopia. For instance, simple television viewing induces some focusing effort and could thrust the susceptible person into myopia.

Prescribing glasses which are somewhat weaker in power than needed for optimum sight does, in selected individuals, have a small retarding effect. The amount is very modest, however, and of no great consequences in the overall picture.

The use of bifocals has proponents because the theory is elegantly simple. On the assumption that the focusing effort at near causes myopia, bifocals should lessen the focusing effort and retard increases. In actual practice it works with some youngsters but not all. The habitual reading distance is probably a big factor. Many nearsighted children who are fitted with bifocals will hold the reading material even closer than before. Reading at eight or ten inches virtually negates the effect of the bifocal—focusing is stimulated and myopia progresses on its merry way. The concept of bifocals would be more effective if the reading material were held at sixteen inches, but try to enforce that. If we could get the child to read at eighteen to twenty-two inches it would be more effective than prescribing bifocals. However, the nearsighted child seems to have a "need" to read very close and "enjoys" the ensuing large image size. This may well be the original reason for the myopia.

Clinical experience indicates that giving bifocals indiscriminately to all is just as wrong as not providing bifocals to those who might benefit. The most successful candidate is the child who can be induced to relax the focusing strain. Foremost in this group is the pseudo-myope for whom bifocals, accompanied by visual therapy, is quite effective. For some obscure reason, girls respond better to bifocals than boys.

Anecdotal reports indicate that the wearing of hard contact lenses is an affective regimen. It's not unusual for youngsters who needed frequent changes in their glasses to require little further changes after switching to contacts. The reasons are not clear and the studies are inconclusive. Some of the factors may be: Corneal curvature changes, pupil size, metabolic changes, alterations in the accommodation-convergence relationship, intraocular pressure changes, corneal thickness, relaxation of focusing spasms, molding effect of the contact lens, anterior chamber depth, etc. With so many possibilities, it is difficult to determine which one or which combination holds the myopia in check. On the other hand, some authorities contend that myopia control through wearing contact lenses is merely an artifact.

Soft contact lenses don't appear to have much influence on myopia reduction. The key reason could be that they do not apply firm pressure on the cornea; the phrase "pressure on the cornea" is an introduction into orthokeratology.

The word is derived from "ortho" meaning zero power, and "keratology" referring to the study of the cornea. According to the practitioners of this speciality, myopia is reduced by the action of contact lenses applying flattening pressure on the cornea. Flattening the cornea counterbalances the excessive light-focusing power of the eye.

Here's the working principal. The front surface of the cornea is measured with instruments or photographically recorded for computer analysis of its curvature. Using this information, the contact lenses are designed to achieve a small, flattening effect. As the cornea's contour changes, different lenses are fitted for additional flattening; the cycle is repeated several times. When the reshaping process is completed and 20/20 sight obtained without the need of any correction, the contact lens wearing time is slowly reduced. If the shape of the cornea has been permanently altered, no further correction is necessary.

However, for most people, if the wearing of contact lenses is completely discontinued, the cornea will tend to resume its original curvature and vision will decline. To prevent this from occurring, "retainer" lenses are fitted to hold the shape of the cornea in check. They are the final lenses (presumably) which will be needed. To maintain their good vision, some people have to wear the retainer lenses six to eight hours a day; some need only wear them a few hours every two or three days; a few rare individuals get by with only a single wearing every few months. The availability of gas permeable lenses makes it conceivable for these contacts to be worn as retainers overnight while sleeping.

The length of the orthokeratology procedure is anywhere from 12 months to three years. Generally, people with low or moderate myopia can expect to obtain satisfactory results; however, some don't respond well at all. For extremely nearsighted persons, the best that can be hoped for is a reduction in the prescription of the correcting lenses. Thus, for high myopia, we consider orthokeratology of dubious value.

Orthokeratology can be a safe and useful tool in myopia reduction if the corneal shape and vision is frequently monitored by a skilled, experienced practitioner. One tremendous advantage of this method over the surgical methods described later is that it can be discontinued at any time without permanent annoying and/or disabling side effects. Surgery is irreversible.

The success of visual therapy in controlling myopia is very difficult to assess. We know with proper training it is possible to relieve the stress of focusing and convergence while reading. It also works well in cases of pseudo-myopia. However, a total program of therapy to halt myopia is another matter. The idea of a six, seven or eight-year-old following a strict therapy routine is hard to swallow. The doctors who claim to have achieved control of nearsightedness by using certain therapy instruments apparently have very obedient young patients or a remarkable facility to command compliance. We cannot envision a high success ratio.

The use of drug therapy to control myopia relies on the principle of avoiding all focusing at near. Drugs are instilled into the eyes to paralyze the focusing mechanism for weeks or months at a time. This method has little to recommend it as it interferes with the development of the child's visual patterns.

The value of proper nutrition can be guessed at, but proof is hard to come by. One body of thought is that the many additives in our processed foods can impact on the development of the nervous tissue of the brain. The eye, being an extension of the brain, might also be affected. The lack of certain critical vitamins and minerals may be a factor. It is safe to suggest that a well balanced diet is healthier overall even if it doesn't reduce myopia.

In the past, surgical intervention to reduce or control myopia has been a risky, last resort venture. In recent years, a corneal surgery technique called Radial Keratotomy has been employed with moderate success (and considerable fanfare).

While the procedure is relatively simple, the results range from excellent to downright bad. The preliminary step is to thoroughly study the cornea for shape, thickness and cell density with computerized instruments. During the operation the surgeon uses a diamond scalpel to make a series of "pie-slice" radial cuts on the cornea, avoiding the center and the fine meshwork of blood vessels at the edge. Since the cornea is only about 0.5 millimeter (1/50th of an inch) thick, extreme care is necessary to avoid cutting too deep. When the cuts heal, the cornea will flatten (as in orthokeratology), resulting in a decrease of nearsightedness. The precise change is fairly predictable in most cases. Although there is generally improvement in sight, some people are aware of annoying side effects such as glare, haze and distortions. As with any operation, serious, unexpected catastrophes are possible and this one is no exception—potential permanent damage can occur.

Even employing a finely honed diamond scalpel the edges of the cuts are not completely smooth which hinders the healing and affects the outcome. Therefore, many surgeons are switching to lasers to gain better control and smoother tissue removal. There is also better predictability in the outcome. (See Chapter 33, Lasers & The Eye.)

You may be a candidate for Keratotomy if you:

1.   Have a normal, disease-free cornea.
2.   Have a small or moderate degree of nearsightedness.
3.   The nearsightedness is fairly stable.
4.   Cannot wear contact lenses.

In spite of its seeming allure, the verdict is not yet in. The most troublesome aspect are the unknown long-range consequences. After all, a perfectly healthy and intact cornea is being tampered with. How will the cornea respond years later to stresses such as injuries, infections, or even normal aging changes? We just don't know. Undoubtedly, with the pace of technology being what it is, it's difficult to predict future surgical methods. Before consenting to any elective surgical corneal procedure consult with your optometrist.

Prevention, control and corneal modification will continue to be debated, and out of those debates some further solutions may emerge. We can anticipate a time in the future when emphasis will be on preventing the onset of myopia through, possibly, genetic engineering. If that seems too "far out", we can, perhaps, discover ways to keep the amount of myopia to a minimum.

VIII

Vision in Sports

30

"Keep Your Eye On The Ball"

Millions of people participate in sports on a regular basis and are always seeking the perfect stance or form, that special new piece of equipment, and that extra winning tip to make them better performers. As you go up the ladder from casual amateur to professional, the quest becomes more intense and the payoffs greater.

There are exercise machines to build up your muscles, foods and vitamins for strength and endurance, psychological counseling to give you a winning attitude, special gloves and shoes to enhance grip and speed, and even designer sport clothes to bolster your ego. Just about every sport has its complements of magazines and books, television shows and videos. If you leaf through the pages or watch your screen you'll come across stories on training programs, nutrition, step-by-step instructions, hypnosis, winning strategies, but rarely will you find much about a very critical ingredient in most sports—vision. That's a glaring oversight since vision is the single biggest factor in directing and controlling your actions and reactions.

Clear Sight Is Not Enough

Most people don't think about vision at all unless glasses or contact lenses are needed to correct sight, and even that consideration is only for keenness of sight. While keen sight is an important attribute, it is just one of many inputs the brain's visual system requires for you to "see." These inputs are processed via numerous, intricate steps, then combined to provide you with a rich and detailed visual scene. The fact that you seem to automatically perceive the scene is silent evidence of the constant and simultaneous information solving process going on in the background. A partial list of what the visual system has to contend with and resolve would include changes in lightness or brightness, color discrimination, following or tracking moving objects, judging size and distance, detecting motion, determining the depth of objects in space, differentiating between self-motion and the motion around you, and recognizing shapes and textures.

All this information processing is mediated by separate subsystems (or channels) and then combined by the brain into a total perception of the visual scene. A critical fact to understand is that some channels require less time, others more time to come to a "decision." For instance, you can detect the movement of an object quicker than you can determine its trajectory or its exact position in space. These working times range from less than 1/100th second to several tenths of a second. While this may seem quite fast, for some high speed sports it may not be fast enough.

To faithfully reproduce our physical world, the subsystems must depend on clear sight from both eyes, good focusing ability, proper and rapid alignment of both eyes, easy and accurate eye movements, precise centering, true feedback signals, correct neural connection, etc.

It is unusual for all the subsystems to work perfectly since aberrations in your visual development during infancy and childhood may warp later functions (a very good reason for a vision examination at an early age). There are also normal, individual variations from one person to the next just as there are for height, strength, reflexes, etc. By and large, most of us can get along adequately unless the visual system is challenged to peak performance as in many sporting activities (although it can also happen during prolonged reading, driving or scrutinizing a video display terminal).

A Challenge to the Visual System

Let's examine the visual task of hitting a baseball. A good major-league fast ball pitch takes about 4/10 second to reach home plate. It takes about 2/10 second for the swinging bat to cross the plate area. Obviously, you can't wait for the ball to cross the plate to start your swing. Therefore, the decision whether to swing or not, and where to swing must be made within 2/10 second of the pitcher's release when the ball is still some 25 feet away. In other words, the visual system must calculate the speed, position, and direction of the ball, then predict its speed and position when crossing the plate 2/10 second later.

A curve ball will take about 6/10 second to reach home plate, but the extra time is well spent trying to predict where the ball will cross the plate, or perhaps miss the strike zone. The decision must be made when the ball is still about 20 feet away. It becomes apparent that if the pitcher can do something to alter the speed or trajectory during those last 20 feet, the batter cannot adjust the swing in time. Assuming contact is made with the ball, the batter has to time that contact to within 1/100 second for the ball to be hit into fair territory. Swinging just a fraction too soon or too late results in a foul ball.

This all sounds very formidable. Yet, batters do hit fast balls, curve balls, change-ups, split-finger fast balls, and even knuckle balls. The explanation is twofold. First, certain visual capabilities are decidedly quicker and more accurate in some individuals. Second, the so-called "guessing" of what the pitcher is going to throw is top-down visual processing in the sense that the brain is primed for seeing a certain pitch. If the guess is correct, the visual processing time is shortened. If the guess is wrong, the batter is "frozen" or badly fooled because reality doesn't conform to what the brain expected—it's a visual illusion condition.

Fortunately for many of us, there are less challenging games, visually speaking. Moderately poor sight, slow information processing, and even some distortions in the visual system should not keep you from running a good race, tackling a fullback, enjoying billiards, or being a respectable bowler. But regardless of the game, wouldn't you enjoy it more if your performance improved? Often the difference is good vision—not just good sight. The remainder of this chapter will attempt to point out the difference.

There is wide range of visual requirements for various sports and games. For archery or pistol shooting you could actually get by very nicely with only one seeing eye. For sky diving good vision isn't all that critical as long as you can enjoy the view and see the approaching ground. If you want to consistently hit the ball in the major leagues, you'd better have excellent binocular vision.

In team sports, visual requirements differ with each player's role. The quarterback has more sophisticated visual needs than the tackle. In baseball, there are more demanding visual requirements for an infielder than an outfielder, and even differences among infield positions.

Non-Action and Action Sports

Let's disregard those activities which require only minimal vision—weight lifting, rowing, jogging, etc., and concentrate on those that require good vision for normal performance. It would be convenient for this discussion to differentiate between non-active (static) and active (dynamic) sports.

In non-active sports, the object and player are stationary. Golf is a good example. The golfer and the ball do not move in relation to each other, thus the visual system is observing a stationary object. Certainly you follow the flight of the ball after you hit it, but his has no bearing on the outcome. (Body English is not really effective.)

In action sports there are four possibilities: (1) only the object is moving. Example: skeet shooting. (2) only the player is moving. Example: bowling. (3) objects and player(s) are moving. Example: racquetball. (4) object and many players (team) are moving. Example: basketball.

In the static golf situation the visual system can leisurely decide exactly where the ball is. (Counter intuitively, an overly long inspection time could actually be a hindrance, as we'll point out later.) In the dynamic racquetball situation, the visual system has to determine in a split second where the ball is in three-dimensional space, and on the basis of some hasty computation, predict where it will be a fraction of a second later. It sounds as if it should be a very complex feat, and it is, yet the visual system of many people does a generally respectable job of it. Is there a secret to any of it?

If you listen to everyone, apparently not. All you have to do is:

"Keep you eye on the ball!!" (Not even both eyes?) This phrase echoes through stadiums, gyms and playing fields. Depending on the sport there are variations such as: "Keep your eye on the puck!" and "Keep you eye on the goal!" There is nothing wrong with the statement, but as with many things in life, it is easier said than done. Let's check out why.

Dynamic Vision

First, let's lay the groundwork. Biological evolution has geared the visual system to respond mostly to motion to provide "early warning radar" for something approaching (or you approaching something) which could be harmful. Static vision is handy for seeing an apple in a tree, or as a stable background against which motion takes place. Research indicates that dynamic vision and static vision are in many ways two separate components of the visual apparatus. Detecting motion is a distinct, very high priority item.

Of course, you realize that eye movement alone (and the eyes are in constant motion) does not impart movement to an object or scene. When you glance around a room, the images of tables and chairs are sweeping across the retina at the back of the eyes in the same manner as when true motion is taking place. But because the brain factors out eye, head and body movements everything appears stationary.

The entire visual process is complicated, many-faceted and far from being fully understood. However, for the purpose of this sports topic, we can illustrate some of the intricacies of dynamic vision with the common experience of a baseball being thrown towards you.

As the baseball begins its flight both eyes have to "lock" onto it. Within about 15/100 second the eyes will make a rapid saccade to pursue and catch up with the speeding ball. A saccade is a quick, ballistic jump of the eyes from one point in space to a predetermined second point. This saccade is usually a little off target and a second, smaller saccade will correct for the undershoot. During a saccade there is almost no input to the visual system—for that brief moment you are "blind" just as you are during a blink. (Amid rapt visual attention the blink rate is reduced to limit that source of interruption.)

The motion-in-depth system and the size judgement system, working from clues in the retinal images, are furiously computing just how far away the ball is and how fast it is closing in. Concurrently, the tracking system keeps the eyes fastened on the ball. As the ball gets closer the eyes have to converge their line of sight to keep the image centered in your view. While all this is going on, other subsystems must provide you with information about shape, texture, color and the entire peripheral scene. (If there's a tree to your right you'd prefer not to lunge in that direction to catch the ball.)

Obviously, it's a very busy time for the visual system and short cuts must be utilized. To do so, the visual system uses limited clues to generate what is seen. Thus, as soon as the trajectory of the ball is established, the trajectory attention tapers off so that other facets can gain concentration. If there is an unexpected subtle position change such as a slightly windblown ball while your eyes are executing a saccade, the visual system will be "blind" to it and you'll "misjudge" the catch. A large change in trajectory such as a tennis ball kicking off the top of the net will put the system back into high gear to repeat all the steps and calculations with the inevitable time delay. Therefore, you may be unable to react quickly enough to the change.

Another source of potential system error is the "anticipatory" saccade. The eyes will frequently execute a saccade in anticipation of where the brain thinks the next point of interest will be. In most cases this saccade is a smart tactic for the visual system which is pressed for time and wants to get a jump on the action. In reading, for instance, it is a very useful time saver. In sports, however, it can be counter productive because you take your eyes of the ball (puck, etc.) a split second before you should. Remember that you are "blind" during the saccade and if you make this involuntary glance before the position-in-depth and speed have been fully computed, you will slightly miscalculate the contact point. A slight miscalculation is all it takes to separate the pros from the semi-pros. The anticipatory saccades vary from person to person. In some the tendency is slight, in others it happens frequently.

As an example of saccades causing problems: On a number of occasions we carefully observed major-league baseball pitchers' eye movements through binoculars. Inevitably, if the pitcher flicked his eyes (a saccade) off the catcher's glove target as he was about to release the ball, the ball would miss the target in the direction of the eyes' flick. It makes good sense. Try hammering a nail and glance to the side just as you are starting your downswing. More often than not you'll miss the nail (and mash your thumb).

There are many timesaving tricks the visual system resorts to, but the ones mentioned are enough to illustrate that keeping your eyes constantly on the ball is practically impossible. Furthermore, contrary to the notion that a very long look would be helpful, the visual system really wants to move on to something else. Conversely, too short a look (less than 1/10 second) will keep some of the subsystems from completing their calculations.

Consider the golfer addressing the ball for 5 or 10 seconds. The visual system is long since bored. It not only reduces its attention but is probably making saccades all over the place. Your best tactic is to think about your swing but to look at the ball (or better still, a detail on the ball) for only the last second. Even that may be too long for some golfers. You might even try looking at a spot on the ground a few inches to the right of the ball (if your swing is from the right) so the inevitable anticipatory saccade will take you to the point of contact instead of away from it. You'll need to experiment a bit with the exact number of inches suitable for your system.

In action sports it is difficult, nearly impossible to avoid anticipatory or spurious eye movements, but here are a few tips:

1. If you're tracking a ball don't just look at the ball but search for any writing or seam on the surface. The concentration needed to scrutinize for detail will usually maintain the visual system's attention.

2. It is easy to be distracted by a moving opponent or teammate. A split-second glance will interrupt the flow of information to the visual system and must be avoided. Even the awareness of the other players will cause some interference, albeit less.

3. Analyze the movements of objects in your particular sport and try to avoid useless, time consuming glances. For example, in tennis most receivers watch the server's ball being tossed up. It is a useless glance because when the ball is suddenly hit by the racket, you can lose 1/10 second switching your visual system from looking up and down to having to track a speeding, approaching ball. It makes more sense to watch the center of the server's racket arcing towards you. This primes the visual system and gives you a head start on the balls' flight. It takes a lot of practice and discipline to avoid watching the ball toss, but eventually you should be able to react quicker to a power serve.

The visual system makes use of many clues and strategies to convert light into a meaningful representation of our surroundings. As with all biological systems there are individual variations and deficiencies. Some are easily measured: sight (20/20, 20/70, etc.), depth perception (from an excellent 20 seconds of arc to none), convergence and focusing, and contrast sensitivity. Unfortunately, all these tests are static and there are precious few tests for dynamic vision. Simply stated, the static abilities are important, but when we deal with action sports, the dynamic abilities will determine the level of performance.

Static visual tests have been used for many decades and have research-backed established norms. We are just beginning to delve into dynamic testing and remediation. What is poor, average or superior motion-in-depth perception? What is poor, average or superior eye pursuit ability? Does the athlete with a normal time of 1/100 second for tracking moving objects have an advantage over an athlete whose normal time is 2/100 second? Which of the dozens of visual subsystems are most important for tennis, for skiing, for soccer?

What You See Is Not Always What You See

To accomplish your intentions, regardless of the sport, you must have good hand-eye or foot-eye coordination. Your vision must guide you to the correct spot in space at exactly the right moment. Why doesn't it always? The hitch is that normal biological fluctuations in addition to peculiarities in your visual system may feed you "false" data at certain times and/or in certain areas of the visual field.

To explain that baffling last statement, think of a wide receiver in football missing an accurately thrown pass. The television announcer will intone: "He should have caught it...the ball was right in his numbers." The coach may mutter: "I keep telling him to look the ball right into his hands."

The player doesn't know what happened except that the football was not quite where he thought it should be at the moment he expected it. If he is uncommonly articulate, has a good knowledge of the visual system, and has read this book, there are a least a dozen reasons he could muster for the scowling coach.

Let's merely skim over the more obvious excuses: "The sun was in my eyes." "The ball came at me out of a confusing background." "The defender's hand blocked my view."

The coach, of course, has heard all these before and is not highly impressed. Suppose, though, the player had said: "My eyes made an involuntary saccade towards the oncoming defender. This caused the image of the ball to be interpreted by my visual system as slightly displaced to one side. When I looked back for the ball it was too close for accurate convergence since it's neural action time is 2/10 second. As you know, coach, I either over- or under-converged which affected my size mediated distance judgement. My position-in-depth channel could not be engaged rapidly enough to be a reliable substitute. Furthermore, since the football came from the left, my visual system is known to generate extra saccades in that quadrant. There is also the possibility that being short of oxygen from running caused a bias of the convergence system affecting parts of the visual field which are "blind" to motion-in-

depth. Consequently, in that split-second moment the only clue
I had was the increasing size of the ball. But since it approached
from the left it was outside the 1.5 degrees of visual angle where
size changes are most effective for exact judgement."

Don't worry about understanding that conversation. Do you
think the coach did? It's a safe bet it will never take place on a
football field. Each point of the imaginary conversation is valid,
but a detailed explanation is outside the scope of this chapter.
The critical point to grasp is that dynamic vision—what the
brain "sees," what you "see"—is a complex interaction of many
subsystems. Any number of irregularities can be enough to cause
a slight miscalculation and error.

Were we unfair in picking on a football player? We could
just as easily have sketched a similar scenario for a baseball
player striking out, a tennis pro making an unforced error, or a
hockey defenseman missing a pass. For that matter, these spo-
radic vision miscalculations befall pilots, bicyclists, drivers, or
whenever the visual system is pressured to make split-second
decisions.

In sports, it isn't only the athlete who is subject to not "seeing" what is really there. Referees, umpires and field judges
can also be duped by a lapse in the visual machinery. The old
adage: "Seeing is believing" may be true, but what you believe
is not always a fact.

Can The Problems Be Corrected?

Now that the problems have been outlined, the logical question
is how do we correct them? One tactic might be to rehabilitate
and improve every function of the visual system—the shotgun
approach. The assumption being that if every part works perfectly the entire system will work perfectly. This could be
done with special prescription glasses, contact lenses, and/or
visual therapy. The drawback to this strategy is that we don't
know all the parts and those we do know of are difficult to
measure and even more difficult to improve.

Another path might be to just improve those functions which
are causing the problem. This opens a closet full of questions.
Which functions are most important for a particular sport? Are
they flawed all the time or only under certain conditions? Has
the person learned to compensate? Can the improvements be

stabilized or will the problem resurface? Will other functions be adversely affected?

The bottom line is that there are no ready answers to dynamic vision rehabilitation, but progress is being made as the visual system's inner workings are being unraveled. Until more is known, there is no substitute for a thorough vision examination with special attention to the way you use your eyes and vision. The least that can be done is to ensure that all input signals—the visual system's link to the external world—are reliable indicators and truly represent the physical world.

One excellent way to ensure superior vision for sports is to keep a close watch on your own visual development during infancy and childhood. Of course, this a tongue-in-cheek statement since you are now past this age. The next best thing is to tell your optometrist about your athletic activities and any consistent problems you're experiencing in one area of play. It may be visually related and subject to some type of aid. However, the best aid will rarely be as good as early intervention and care would have been.

If you're a parent, does that trigger some wake-up call about your children? After all, their visual welfare is in your control.

31

Eye Safety In Sports

The number of people in the United States who are engaged in some form of sport activity is quite substantial. Care to guess which activity ranks as the most popular with both men and women? A survey taken a couple of years ago revealed that swimming is number one. In second and third place for men was bicycling and fishing; for women, exercise (including aerobic dancing) and bicycling. Skiing and soccer, which are well down on the list, have been gaining rapidly.

Whatever sport or recreational activity happens to be your favorite, glasses or contact lenses can be fitted to make your participation more enjoyable and safe. If you normally wear glasses, you should not assume that your athletic activity will require the same prescription. To obtain clear, comfortable sight for sports you may need a modified prescription, special lens centering or positioning, tints to remove glare or reflections, bifocals for viewing specific distances or placed in unusual positions, scratch resistant coated plastic, or ultraviolet protection for outdoors.

Contact lenses, rather than glasses, may be the ideal solution for your special needs.

Let's discuss the most popular activity first—swimming. Recreational swimming in a pool merely for exercise hardly requires any sight correction at all. Unless your sight is extremely poor, there is no problem. If you do your swimming in the form of snorkeling or scuba diving, you want good sight. Your prescription can be bonded into swim goggles or the diving mask, or you can wear contact lenses under either the goggles or mask.

Bicycling poses no unusual requirements except for the safety aspect which will be discussed later. Fishing may require some special tinted lenses, also discussed later. Exercise programs such as weight lifting or aerobic dancing do not depend on good sight. However, if your exercise is in the form of gymnastics, good sight is quite important and soft contact lenses are the choice.

Actually, the choice for most sports is soft contact lenses provided they can be made up in your prescription. The benefits of soft contacts are greater the more active and competitive an athlete you are. The advantages are much more than merely cosmetic. For one thing, there is a wider field of view which is very important in games such as soccer, hockey, basketball, etc. If you've ever been annoyed by glasses which steam up when you perspire or which insist on slipping down your nose, contacts can be the answer. Furthermore, with contacts there is no distortion of the field of vision when you look to the sides as when you look through the sides of your glasses. Finally, soft contacts will rarely slip off the eye or allow dust to get underneath the lens.

Hard contact lenses have most of these advantages except for the last two—they can slip off and particles can get underneath. However, the vision is often crisper and less subject to slight variations. The variations (caused by the soft lens drying or buckling) might possibly interfere at a critical moment, such as when a baseball hitter watches a pitched ball.

The middle-aged or older person who normally wears bifocals may discover that some sports are not very compatible with the bifocals. For example, if you are a golfer, you know that the reading segment gets in the way when you address the ball.

One solution is to have glasses with only a distance correction, although keeping score on the scorecard can become an ordeal. A better solution is to have bifocals made with the reading segment placed very low or to the side. Then you can see the ball as well as the score. A more imaginative solution might be bifocal contact lenses which provide both far and near sight. Bifocal contact lenses might also be very useful for hunters, card players, etc. Check out the possibility with your optometrist.

Tinted Lenses for Sports

If your sport takes you outdoors, tinted lenses can enhance your ability to see and will reduce eyestrain and fatigue. Good quality sunglasses with the proper color and darkness can offer relief from excessive glare, reduce overhead brightness and cut reflection dazzle from water or snow. Even on a hazy, slightly overcast day, the light scattering effect of the atmosphere makes the use of tinted lenses useful.

It's an easy matter to control the amount and quality of light entering the eye by tinting the lens, polarizing the light, using photochromic glass which darkens in sunlight, mirror coating the lenses, or combining several of these techniques.

For the average sunlit, outdoor conditions, a grey sunglass which absorbs 70% to 85% of the light is preferable. If your sport takes you out on the water, beach, desert, or snow, use a dark grey, polarized lens that absorbs 80% to 95% of the light.

If you are one of millions who enjoy fishing, you spend a great deal of time on lakes and rivers. The sun reflecting off the water's surface can cause almost painful glare. Why don't you have your prescription made up into polarizing sunglasses? They will eliminate just about all the glare and even permit you to see below the surface of the water.

The hunter who spends a great deal of time in forests should not exceed a 50% light reduction even on a bright day, and not more than 25% on an overcast day. Probably the best way to accomplish this is with the use of the changeable photochromic lenses.

Whenever only overhead glare is a problem, a gradient type of tinting (dark on top and fading to clear at the bottom) can be useful. Or perhaps you need a double gradient tinting with the center lighter than the top and bottom. Obviously, there are many possibilities and a single pair of glasses will not solve every lighting condition you may encounter.

To be really up-to-date, you could get tinted soft contact lenses in a variety of colors. You could then choose the color suitable for the prevailing light conditions provided it isn't exceptionally bright.

Some tennis players benefit from a light yellow or gold tint when playing indoors or on a cloudy day. It seems to make the ball easier to track by brightening the background. This also applies to other games where similar conditions exist, although not all players appreciate an improvement.

Eye Safety in Sports

Let's describe an encounter that could happen to you. You've had a hard, frustrating day at the office and you're looking forward to unwinding with a racquetball game. Your opponent is quite aggressive and after some rallies, the game is developing into a fine contest. You make a great shot on a serve return and whirl to follow the ball. Suddenly, something seems to explode in your eye and searing pain shoots through your head. You realize that you've been hit in the eye by either the ball or your opponent's racket.

If you're relatively lucky it may only be a cut eyebrow; if you're not, it could be as serious as loss of sight in the eye. Whether minor or major, the injury could easily have been avoided by wearing proper safety glasses. Of course, you are not alone.

Thousands of children and adults suffer eye injuries every year as a result of playing racket sports, hockey, and soccer without any eye protection or with inadequate protection. Inadequate protection can mean wearing your everyday spectacles, improper safety eyewear, or lensless eyeguards.

The small, hard racquetball can reach speeds of 130 mph, a hockey puck sometimes travels too fast for the eyes to track, and even the simple badminton bird can reach high velocities for the first 10 feet of travel. Besides these projectiles, eye injuries can also be caused by game equipment (bats, hockey sticks, rackets), and opponents (fingers, knees). Yet very few people wear eye protection. It's the automobile seat belt syndrome—injuries happen to other people, not to you.

What types of eye injuries can be sustained? They range from a simple abrasion to a completely lacerated eyeball. The more serious injuries can include massive hemorrhage, a dislocated eye lens, cataract formation, retinal detachment, or blowout fracture of the thin bones of the orbit. Even if there is not total sight loss, there may not be complete vision recovery.

Suitable Safety Eyewear

The type of safety eyewear suitable for you will depend on the sports you're engaged in. The sports most likely to cause injuries are those which use high speed projectiles, some type of implements, or attain great speeds. These would include rifle shooting, hockey, motorcycling, skiing, racquetball, baseball, tobogganing, etc. Safety eyeglasses or goggles should be worn in all these activities. Just about any sport can be dangerous for children because of their inexperience and slower reactions.

If you or your children are involved in hazardous sports, we assume you're concerned enough to use the best possible eye protection. The choice lens material for safety glasses is polycarbonate plastic. The frame should be made of a special safety material and be specially designed for the sport.

Lenses made of polycarbonate are able to withstand tremendous impact without shattering or breaking—they're as tough as steel. Despite the strength, however, they can be scratched and exhibit some color aberrations. Both of these characteristics can be effectively reduced with a chemical coating applied to the surfaces of the lenses.

Safety frames are made of a material able to withstand and absorb shock without breaking into fragments. The lenses are held in place by extra deep grooves so that they cannot be forced out into the eye, face, etc. The hinges are well secured and positioned to avoid being forced into the skin. You'll be able to keep the glasses in a proper position much easier if the temples wrap around your ears.

Since ordinary, everyday glasses do not have these safety attributes, you can appreciate the risk of wearing them during hazardous sports. If you require glasses to see clearly, there are three ways to ensure safety:

1. Wear safety goggles that fit over your glasses.
2. Have your prescription made up into safety glasses.
3. Have prescription lenses bonded into a safety goggle.

In less dangerous sports such as bicycling and volleyball, regular plastic lenses which have been made scratch-resistant and mounted in a safety frame should serve quite well. The key is the use of a safety frame, since a regular frame will rarely survive a strong blow or collision. Rimless frames, very stylish for regular wear, should be avoided for athletics. The frames easily move out of alignment and the lenses can be popped loose. A solid metal frame is all right if it has a molded, one-piece bridge. The separate, adjustable nosepad-type frame can lacerate the nose if jammed against the face.

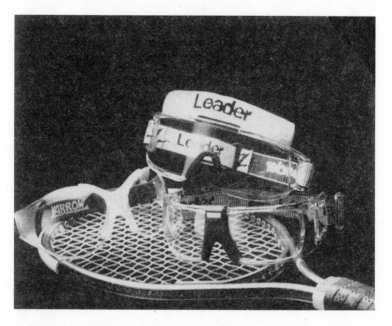

Both prescription and non-prescription sport glasses are available in a wide range of styles and colors.

There is one more safety aspect to consider, and that is the possibility of the lenses fogging up and obscuring your sight. Skiers, ice skaters, and motorcyclists, among others, are susceptible to this problem. Your best bet is goggles with anti-fog double lenses separated by an air space. Otherwise, you may choose goggles with a tiny built-in fan or with vents on the sides.

There is proper safety eyewear available for every sport and game. Check with your eye care professional. There isn't a reason in the world why you should be playing Russian roulette every time you go out to enjoy your activity, or have to worry every time your kids are involved in theirs.

IX

Vision, Computers and Lasers

32

How To Deal With Your Video Display Terminal

The use of computers with their video display terminals (VDTs) in business offices and in homes has become prodigious. With so many people involved in working at these VDTs, it's no wonder there are so many voiced apprehensions and complaints.

The apprehension centers around possible harm from radiation emitted by the monitors. There are conflicting scientific studies as to the validity of the dangers. Some very weak X-rays are given off by the terminals (less than 1% of safety levels) but manufacturers are doing a better job of shielding in the newer machines. The other area of concern involves electromagnetic radiation (EMR) which is given off by all electric devices including your toaster, television, etc. There may be a difference in the amount of time spent near the toaster as compared to near the terminal which is what worries some people. Actually, the radiation is energetic over only a short range, so moving a little further away from the monitor (20 inches) might be a prudent step. It'll probably be years before any final scientific determination is made.

The complaints commonly heard are based on symptoms which fall into two categories—general and/or visual. The general complaints are: headaches at the back of the head, pains in the neck, aching shoulders, sore back, and painful wrists. Visual symptoms include: difficulty in fixating on the words, blurred or double vision, tender and aching eyes, headaches above the eyes, glare sensitivity, and burning, red eyes.

Let's examine the general complaints first. They are all related to the environmental conditions and the placement of the VDT, desk, chair, etc. The key to maintaining comfort is total flexibility of all components; i.e., everything should be adjustable. The chair height and back support, the keyboard, the distance and height of the screen, etc. If we were to pick one item that is frequently at fault it is a screen that is too high. Time and again the VDT is simply plunked on top of the computer cabinet making it necessary to constantly raise the head which stresses the neck vertebrae causing pain. The top of the screen should be BELOW eye level. Making this simple adjustment will often relieve those neck pains and headaches. While it sounds simple, the work stations are sometimes so badly designed that it's just not possible to lower the VDT. If you can lower the screen be sure it doesn't get so low and with an exaggerated upward tilt that it picks up overhead reflections. (More about reflections later.) The ideal distance to the screen for most people is about 22 inches.

The lettering on the screen should have a good resolution. You may or may not be able to control the colors, but you should at least experiment with the contrast level to find one that seems most suitable. Monochromatic monitors with green or amber letters seem to please most people. If you have a color monitor, try some different combinations. Generally, the best partnership of letters to background are colors which are next to each other in the rainbow. (If you've forgotten the rainbow distribution is violet, blue, green, yellow, orange, red). Conversely, red on blue is quite annoying because these colors focus well apart in the eyes; both cannot be in clear focus at the same time. Definitely try a white or a black as one of the choices.

The visual symptoms are more difficult to deal with. The first thing to check for and eliminate is any reflections off the surface of the screen—even small ones are very annoying to the visual system. Reflections could be caused by ceiling lights, windows, or a desk lamp somewhere above or behind you. The best way to test for this is to turn the VDT off and see if there are any reflected images on the screen. If there are, you can locate the source by holding a mirror in front of the screen. Then angle the screen to remove the reflections or shade the window and/or light. If neither remedy is possible, you can fit an anti-reflective filter over the screen.

Another common source of annoyance is a light shining directly into your eyes from an unshaded window or fixture. This must be eliminated or you'll have to squint your eyes, causing great discomfort. If you wear glasses the effect could be worse because of reflections within your lenses, although this is easy to rectify. Tinting the lenses and/or a darker tint at the top of the lenses combined with an anti-reflective coating should help quite a bit.

The general illumination in an office where VDTs are used should be lower than in a regular office. Indirect illumination is best with the ceilings brighter than the walls.

If, after doing all these things, you are still experiencing eye and vision problems, a visit to your optometrist is in order. Before you go, measure the distance from the screen to your eyes and the distance to other reading matter. The doctor will conduct additional tests and evaluate your vision for your working distance. Even if you normally don't need glasses, you may require a prescription just for viewing the screen. Then again, your regular-wear glasses may have to be modified for your work. This applies particularly to bifocal wearers. The type, power and placement of the reading portion often has to be changed from what you might normally use. It may turn out that you would be best off with a trifocal or progressive bifocal. It should not surprise you if a pair of glasses has to be made which is specifically dedicated to your work. It's a matter of having the right tool for the job.

33

Lasers and The Eye

Shortly after lasers were invented in 1960, the first medical applications to benefit from the unique qualities of laser light was the treatment of eye conditions. It makes sense because the transparent cornea allows light (regular and laser) to freely enter the inside of the eye. Steady progress in laser development and medical treatment has been made in the past quarter century. The decade of the 90s will surely see some provocative and interesting extensions of the laser's use in eye care.

A very short and simplified primer on lasers is in order at this point. The word laser is an acronym for Light Amplification by Stimulated Emission of Radiation. It means the light is made to behave in a precise, orderly course rather than in its usual random fashion. The sun or a light bulb shines at many wavelengths (colors) which combine to create what we see as "white" light, plus non-visible radiation. The light disperses in all directions much as a crowd of people in a park stroll about randomly. On the other hand, laser light is limited to a narrow wavelength in one corresponding direction like a column of precision-marching soldiers.

Three elements are needed to create such a uniform beam of light: a suitable source of excitable atoms, a way to excite the atoms, and a feedback mechanism. The source material can be a gas, liquid or solid. An electric current or flash lamp is the usual means employed to excite the atoms to a higher energy level. The excited state lasts less than one thousandth of a second, and a photon is spontaneously released when the atom returns to its normal energy level. A photon is an elementary particle of electromagnetic radiation. Some of these photons will strike other energized atoms, resulting in identical-wavelength photons traveling in the same direction. This process is repeated over and over again with the vast number of available atoms creating a cascade of photons.

The feedback mechanism consists of two parallel mirrors at each end of the containment tube. One mirror is totally reflective, the other partially transmissive. The photons sweep back and forth between the mirrors; each sweep intensifies the lasing effect. When the intensity reaches a critical level, the laser light beam emerges from one end through a partially transmissive mirror. Because the beam is coherent (in perfect step) it is very narrow and can be easily focused to a tiny spot.

Selectively choosing the "fuel" material stored in the laser tube determines the wavelength output of the laser. Most often, this is in the ultraviolet, visible light or infrared regions. The amount of power output is governed by the excitable material and the potency and duration of energy delivered to it. Laser beams can be continuous or pulsed in short bursts. Controlling all these variables creates a variety of laser beams with a range of performances.

PHOTOCOAGULATION: The earliest use relied on the simple conversion of the laser energy into heat. Since various parts of the eye absorb different wavelengths, the laser action can be concentrated fairly exclusively on the selected tissue or cells. Photocoagulation occurs when the temperature is high enough, about 65°C (150°F), to alter proteins. It is commonly used to "tack down" the edges of a retinal tear to the underlying tissue, to stop the bleeding from retinal hemorrhages, and to destroy retinal blood vessels sprouting out of control in diabetics.

PHOTOVAPORIZATION: If the temperature is raised above 100°C (212°F), the boiling point of water, photovaporization takes place—the water in the tissues is vaporized. In practice, a temperature of about 400°C (750°F) is used to kill off malignant tumor cells.

PHOTOCHEMICAL effects can be produced with appropriate lasers. One type of dye laser will photoradiate and kill tumor cells after they have been sensitized with special drugs.

PHOTOABLATION involves the use of pulses of UV radiation to break tissue molecules. This is being used for reshaping the cornea to eliminate sight disorders.

PHOTODISRUPTION is a technique using incredibly short bursts (less than 10 one-millionth of a second) of near-infrared light to create a very high temperature (over 10,000°C) which strips electrons from atoms. In effect, it separates tissue like a tiny scalpel. This is represented by the popular YAG laser used to destroy the cloudy lens capsule, the so-called "second cataract" which can develop after cataract surgery.

Diagnostic Uses

There are a number of laser instruments which have been (and are being) developed to diagnose and measure various eye and vision functions.

INTERFEROMETER: A laser interferometer makes use of high contrast interference fringes (black and white stripes) focused into an eye with poor sight. The poor sight could be from a cataract or amblyopia and the test results will reasonably predict the recoverable sight after treatment.

VELOCIMETER: The laser doppler velocimeter gauges the blood flow in the retinal blood vessels. A new concept is to use a modified version to measure the exact distances inside the eye. This will eventually replace ultrasonography in determining the prescription power of a lens implant after a cataract removal.

Another novel idea is to use a laser to quantify the concentration of proteins that cause cataracts. It's very important for people who are taking drugs which might have a cataract-forming side effect. The information would be available long before any clinical signs of cataracts are noticed.

Therapeutic and Refractive Uses

A very common use is to perform a capsulotomy after cataract surgery. Part of the capsule of the eye's lens is left in place as a holding platform for the lens implant. (See Chapter 30.) Unfortunately, many times the capsule will become as cloudy as the original cataract. Before lasers, a surgical procedure was required to enter the eye and cut the capsule away. With the laser, the intense laser beam virtually "explodes" the cloudy tissue into microscopic debris so that sight is restored. But sometimes this will create additional complications because the debris can clog the trabecular meshwork, a narrow belt of sieve-like tissue within the eye through which natural eye fluid is drained. If clogged, the pressure in the eye can very rapidly reach dangerously high levels and cause glaucoma damage.

For persons with narrow-angle glaucoma, another longtime use has been in "burning" a small hole in the iris to relieve the fluid pressure associated with that disease. This becomes necessary if medication is not successful. It's not unusual for the small hole to be become clogged within a year and have to be reopened. A newer, promising procedure uses a laser to enlarge the openings in the trabecular meshwork to enhance the normal drainage. A laser can also be used to reduce the fluid secretion.

Lasers are extremely useful for stabilizing several retinal diseases and conditions. In diabetics, the small blood vessels on the retina may hemorrhage and leak fluid; at a later stage there will be a prolific and haphazard multiplication of blood vessels. These vessels are very fragile, break easily and bleed into the eye. A laser beam can destroy such alien vessels.

A tear or hole in the retina is kept from getting larger by aiming a series of laser pulses around the hole. (These pulses are measured in millionths or billionths of a second.) The heat generated at each tiny spot causes the retina to "weld" to the underlying tissue. A similar technique is used to reduce swelling from leaking blood vessels behind the retina which is a common cause of age related degeneration. The objective is to prevent additional areas from being separated. Unfortunately, if the degeneration is at the macula (the area of sharpest sight), the laser pulses cannot be aimed too close to the macula or they can do more damage than good.

Principally, the advantages of laser surgery over knife surgery are: better precision, no disturbance to adjacent tissue, no need for general anesthesia, and quicker recovery time. Also, some of the laser eye surgeries are just not possible any other way.

What's Ahead

The use of lasers to reshape the cornea and eliminate or reduce nearsightedness, farsightedness and astigmatism is on the horizon. The goal is to supplant a surgical procedure known as radial keratotomy (RK) which has been in limited use for a few years. Using an Excimer laser which removes the cells by decomposition (ablation) instead of a blade keeps the edges smooth and seems to avoid some of the earlier complications.

Ablation by the Excimer laser should also prove beneficial in clearing away a pterygium which is a growth of tissue across the cornea. Another future use of the Excimer laser is in smoothing injury-scarred corneas to restore the even surface and to remove certain types of tumors.

In the area of diagnosis, a scanning laser can be coupled to a television monitor to provide real-time video images of the inside of the eye. This could be advantageous for fluorescein angiography or other health assessments.

It appears that during the next decade, various types of lasers will supplant the surgeon's knife in many ways and will change numerous current testing procedures.

X

Vision Problems of the Aged

34

The Vision of the Aging

merica is a youth oriented society geared to movement, opportunity and vitality. For the older person, whether retired or not, there is the prospect of uncertainty, economic insecurity, and above all, the outlook for declining health. It's harsh enough to be plagued with arthritis, hypertension, elevated cholesterol, diabetes, or a legion of other possible maladies, but when vision goes bad, the fear of blindness and losing one's independence can become a constant worry.

Many of the changes in vision can be considered a function of "normal" aging; others are not. Cataracts, which are by far the single biggest cause for potential sight loss, are so common that they can almost be considered normal. (The next chapter deals entirely with cataracts.)

"Normal" Aging Changes

Even if you manage to avoid the more serious ailments, there are gradual, subtle changes to live with. For instance, the pupil opening gets smaller with age and restricts the amount of light entering the eye. Also, little by little the crystal-clear lens of the eye becomes yellow/brown and loses transparency, acting like a camera filter to absorbs light. This considerably reduces the amount and color purity of light reaching the retina. Additionally, while earlier in life the retinal photoreceptors (rods and cones) are packed tightly together, the density decreases so there are fewer cells which can respond to the available light. All these factors combine for the startling statistic that an 80-year-old person needs *10 times more* light to see the same as a 25-year-old.

The eye's ability to adapt to darkness and recover from bright light gets progressively more meager with age. Color vision and night vision suffer the most since both depend on good quality illumination. Let's put it this way: Older men should have little challenge seeing a woman in a bikini on a bright, sunlit beach, but it might present some trouble at night.

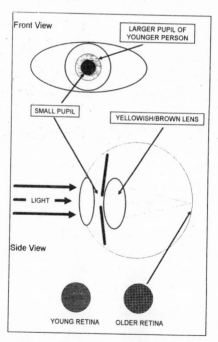

A diagramatic view of why the older eye needs much more light to see. (1) The pupil is smaller, (2) less light gets through the semi-transluscent lens and (3) the photosensitive cells of the retina are not packed as tightly together.

There's more. The vitreous (the gel-like substance filling the inside of the eye) becomes somewhat liquefied with age, making "floaters", "threads" and "flies" more noticeable. These annoying but generally harmless spots cannot be removed. Another annoyance is seeing flashes of light to the extreme sides when the slackened vitreous tugs on the retina.

Watering and Tearing/Dry Eyes

One of the most frequent complaints from older patients concerns watering and tearing of the eyes. There are three probable reasons and they often go together. First, with aging the eyes tend to grow drier as the tear-producing glands in the lids become less efficient and the tears evaporate quickly. As the eyes dry, extra tearing is triggered from wind, dry heat, smoke, etc., which may make it seem to be a wet eye. Second, with aging the lids lose some of their muscle tone and no longer rest flush against the eyeball. Therefore, the tears which normally are drained into the nose through a tiny tube at the inner corner of the lids, well up and spill over. Finally, it is also possible for the tear drainage tube or its opening to become blocked causing the tears to spill over. If that is the reason for the excessive watering, a fairly simple procedure is used to remove the blockage.

Dry eyes will cause burning and a gritty sensation. If you suspect that you have dry eyes, especially in the winter "heating" season, humidifying the air could be beneficial.

Sometimes, the patient may complain of watery eyes, but careful questioning reveals that tears do not actually run down the cheeks. It may be that developing cataracts, macular degeneration or other changes may mimic the visual effects of teary eyes.

Age-Related Macular Degeneration

The macula is that tiny area of the retina which is the most sensitive for seeing fine details. To see something clearly you automatically maneuver your eyes so that the image falls onto the macula and, more specifically, the even tinier, central fovea. Being brain/nerve tissue, the entire retina is immensely sensitive to any reduced blood flow and/or blood leakage. If it occurs at the macula it will bring about a loss of visual acuity which can range from only mild to quite severe. Macular degeneration is the leading causes of poor sight in the elderly.

If the problem is a leaking blood vessel, it may be possible to use laser treatment to seal off the offending vessel provided it isn't too close to the fovea. (See Chapter 33 Lasers.) If the problem is poor circulation, there is no direct treatment. However, there is some evidence that dietary zinc supplements and anti-oxident vitamins may be beneficial in minimizing the sight loss.

Skin Changes

With general skin aging, the lids become loose and baggy which can lead to the eyelashes turning inward or outward. Inward turning lids can irritate the cornea although it may cause only minor distress since corneal sensitivity is diminished with age. The loss of lid muscle tone can also cause the upper lid to droop—senile ptosis (the p is silent). Unless it actually blocks your sight, it is only of cosmetic concern. If the sagging lids are annoying, they can be held up with a fine, flexible wire attached to glasses (ptosis crutch), or lid muscle surgery can be performed.

Medications

Not many individuals savor the "golden" years without taking some medications. If you are, you should know their side effects. Many will precipitate vision effects such as blur, color vision changes, double vision, night blindness, etc. (See Chapter 44.)

Doctors should never be too busy to properly diagnose, then reassure older patients about any particular complaint. When the time is taken to carefully explain the condition, it is easier for people to cope with the ailment; to accept and live with its limitations.

Glaucoma

Glaucoma, much less common than cataracts but more serious (1 to 2% of the population), usually results from poor drainage of the fluid circulating within the eyeball. In the sense that the obstructed drainage is generally the consequence of ongoing aging changes, older people are much more at risk. Since fluid cannot be compressed, too much fluid in the eye will exert pressure rearward. The brunt of the pressure comes to bear on the tiny blood vessels and sensitive nerve fibers at the back of the eye. The usual, chronic (open angle) glaucoma is an insidious, slow-paced process without any obvious symptoms to the person for a long time. If left untreated, side vision will gradually be lost until only a small central area of sight remains.

There is an uncommon type of <u>acute</u> glaucoma which strikes suddenly, accompanied by pain, redness, blurry vision and nausea. Immediate treatment to reduce the pressure is the only way to save sight.

If you have been diagnosed as having the typical chronic type of glaucoma, you are probably using drops and/or oral medication to reduce the fluid pressure. Those who use drops may notice that their vision is adversely affected. If it is, make sure you're not involved in any activity such as driving which requires clear vision. While drops are generally effective in controlling glaucoma, with some people they may, unfortunately, contribute to the development of cataracts.

Glaucoma can also be a secondary complication from other eye conditions or injuries.

Diabetes

Diabetes can strike at any age but as a rule the visual complications will materialize later in life because it has a cumulative affect. A diabetic who is not under control or who "cheats" with the diet or medication is risking sight loss. The major adverse effect is on the tiny blood vessels at the back of the eye which can become blocked, hemorrhage, or grow in wild profusion. This is known as diabetic retinopathy, fast becoming a leading cause of blindness. Laser treatment is often successful in curbing this grave condition. Diabetics are also more likely to develop cataracts.

During a routine eye examination the doctor can detect diabetic changes such as micro-aneurysms (blood vessel ballooning), and dot hemorrhages. These changes actually occur throughout the body, but are most easily discovered in the eyes. Sometimes the patient is not even aware of the diabetic condition, although the disease can be present for many years before visible ocular signs appear.

Diabetics should be mindful of the following:
1. Rapid changes in sight or reading difficulties over a period of a few days or weeks. This is usually caused by fluctuating and high blood sugar levels.
2. Sudden appearance of many spots and "flies" when looking against a bright background. This is often a sign of a hemorrhage or retinal detachment.
3. Hazy or distorted areas in the field of view. This can be caused by tissue swelling from fluid leakage out of the blood vessels.

Hardening of Arteries/High Blood Pressure/Stroke

An all too frequent sequel to blood vessel changes is a stroke (CVA—cerebrovascular accident). A stroke is a sudden and critical impairment to some part of the brain because of an interruption in the blood supply from a blockage or a hemorrhage. You can think of the former as a chunk of dirt which blocks fuel from getting to an auto engine; the latter as a broken fuel line. In the blood stream the "chunk of dirt" is an embolus, a fragment of material which lodges against the walls of the blood vessel and stops the flow. The incidence of strokes is higher after the age of 40 and doubles with every decade of life. Men are much more susceptible at all ages. The single biggest risk factor for a stroke is high blood pressure, followed in order by high cholesterol, smoking, and diabetes.

If a stroke hits that part of the brain involved with vision, you may see flashing or sparkling lights followed by a partial blackout of sight in the affected eye (or both eyes). This frightening situation can last 2 to 15 minutes before sight returns. The "blindness" can be total or only in one sector of the visual field.

Another possibility is that the stroke will affect the control mechanism which points the two eyes to a common target. This will create double vision which may last a few days, weeks, months or the rest of your life. Special prism glasses can be made to compensate for or ease the problem.

While a stroke is a very dramatic episode, narrowed or partly blocked blood vessel can just degrade the normal blood flow to the brain. This reduced supply is called ischemia (is- key-meah). Long standing ischemia of the eyes may cause a sequence of grave eye damaging effects.

An embolus can circulate until it blocks the very tiny blood vessels in the eye itself or a hemorrhage may occur within the eye. Sight loss will quickly follow. These damaging events can be observed by the doctor when looking into the eye. A stroke cannot be seen in the eye.

Recommendations

The passing years are not kind to the eyes and visual system, but there are some things which can minimize the adverse effects.

Good general health is number 1 for good vision. As was mentioned above, maintaining proper blood pressure, keeping cholesterol levels down, not smoking, will all help the visual system retain reasonably good functioning.

Obviously, if you need to wear glasses, do so. Increase the light in your home but keep it evenly bright without glare spots. If possible, try to avoid rapid changes in light levels. You shouldn't expect to come in from bright sunlight and instantly see in a dimly lighted area. Therefore, it is very beneficial to wear sunglasses outdoors to partially offset such quick shifts in illumination. On the other hand, tinted lenses at night or in dark interiors are detrimental because they can further reduce the limited light reaching the retina.

Driving at night on unfamiliar, dark roads should generally be avoided. If you must drive at night, it's a good idea to have an anti-reflective coating applied to your glasses. This will at least eliminate the reflections off the lenses and make it a little easier to see the road and potential hazards.

Is it necessary to state that annual eye examinations are vital? With so many possible potential health problems, it should be very apparent. The examination and diagnosis of most health-related vision problems is reimbursed by Medicare, though routine eyeglasses are not.

35

Cataracts, Cataract Surgery

The most common ailment of the eye which can ultimately lead to loss of sight is the cataract. There's a popular misconception that a cataract is a growth or film over the eyes. Not at all. It is a condition in which the lens within the eye (just behind the colored iris and the pupil) slowly changes its composition from clear and transparent to become cloudy, spotty and opaque. When that happens it's like to trying to see through a steamed-up and/or paint-splattered window pane.

To understand cataract formation, you have to know a little about the lens within the eye. It is responsible for focusing images onto the retina by changing its shape. Biologically, the lens has a very high protein concentration which makes it very susceptible to chemical and electromagnetic radiation (elaborated below). A second important factor—the lens continues to grow throughout life. Think of it as an onion with additional outer layers being added all the time. The early central layers, with no place to go, get more and more compressed and the lens gradually loses some of its pliability. This becomes very evident when you need reading glasses or bifocals in your mid-forties. As the compression continues, the lens becomes yellowish/brown and absorbs more light which both diminishes the amount, and somewhat changes color quality reaching the retina. Perhaps from lack of nutrition reaching the inner layers, linked with other factors (free radicals?), the protein molecules become unstable, the cells lose their transparency and cloudy spots and regions develop.

The rate of clouding is not predictable nor the same in both eyes. One eye may even remain relatively clear. Unlike a totally steamed-up window, the haze is not evenly distributed and the lens may have opaque spots mixed with clear areas. How much vision you retain depends on the size, location, and density of the cloudy patches.

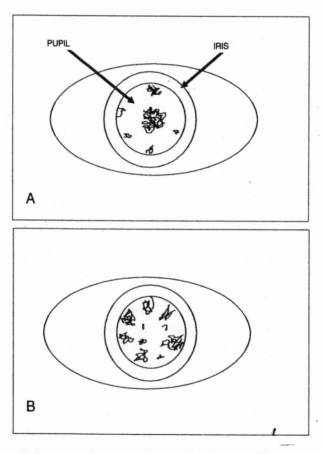

CATARACTS.:*Diagramatic representation of 2 types of cataracts looking into the eye through a dilated pupil. (A) A small central, dense cataract. This could have been caused by long-term use of prednisone for treatment of rheumatoid arthritis. (B) The typical senile (aging) cataract is denser at the periphery and may allow reasonable sight to be retained for years.*

Cataracts usually develop slowly—we are talking about years. We have often watched patients with small opacities that hardly change over a ten year span. Conversely, we have seen a few patients with cataracts that have developed in a few months.

While the effects of oral drugs and diets to retard cataract development are being investigated, there is no current effective prevention treatment. One recent study seems to indicate that nonsteroidal anti-inflammatory drugs such as aspirin or acetaminophen may retard or delay the onset of cataracts. Another study points to vitamin E as possibly effective, but only if daily doses are taken starting as early as age 40. One cataract-retarding drug is awaiting FDA approval.

We are not entirely sure why some people get cataracts, or why they develop on different time scales. We suppose that heredity, nutrition and environmental components are at work, but the mix is not established. Certainly, long term exposure to sunlight (ultraviolet radiation) will adversely affect protein molecules, and adds a strong argument for UV protection. (See Sunglasses and Tinted Lenses.) There are also cataracts which result from eye injuries, diseases and some medications. The most implicated medications are: corticosteroids taken for a long time, and anti-psychotic drugs such as phenothiazines in large doses.

It is quite easy for the optometrist to monitor the progress of your cataract with regular office visits. The visits will also include eye pressure tests and retinal inspections. As the cataract progresses, new glasses will have to be prescribed on a more frequent basis to keep up with your changing vision. Many patients complain of glare. It's caused by scattering of light off the cataract inside the eye. This can be quantified with a brightness acuity test. Tinted lenses are often helpful. If the point is ever reached when a cataract seriously interferes with your sight, it can be removed surgically.

Ophthalmic surgeons have made tremendous strides in cataract surgery in the last decade. The surgery itself is less traumatic on the eye, and replacing the natural lens with an artificial intraocular lens (IOL) implant makes the postoperative sight generally quite good.

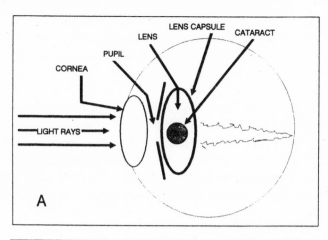

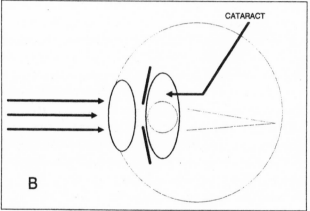

CATARACTS. *The position and density of the cataract will greatly influence how much it effects sight. In this highly diagramatic view, (A) shows a small central, dense cataract which severely interferes with sight. (B) is a much larger but peripheral outside the pupil area. Sight is only mildly affected.*

We won't go into complete details of the operation, just enough information to give you an understanding of what is done in the most often performed procedure. For easier under standing think of the cataractous lens as a small, flattened grape.

The Cataract Surgery

A tiny incision is made in the white of the eye adjacent to the cornea. Through this opening a small tool is inserted to peel off the front of the lens (removing part of the skin of the grape) to expose the cataract (inside of the grape). Then the cataract is bombarded with ultrasound vibrations through a small probe to reduce it to tiny particles—emulsify it; phacoemulsification. A tiny vacuum tube withdraws the emulsified material. A plastic substitute lens (IOL) is slid into place in the pocket formed by the leftover lens capsule (grape skin.) The required dioptric power of the plastic lens has been determine previously by ultrasound or laser. After most surgeries the incision is sutured closed. Sometimes a "stitchless" method is employed. The entire procedure takes about 20 to 30 minutes and is done on an outpatient basis.

Sounds pretty simple, and usually everything works out quite well. However, anytime you get involved with a surgical procedure on individuals who are older and probably not in top physical condition, there are risks and chances of complications.

The primary risk is undergoing a cataract operation when there are other eye conditions or diseases present. Glaucoma, macular degeneration and diabetic retinopathy are the more usual companions to cataracts, and the benefit/risk has to be carefully evaluated. As an example, it may be necessary to remove the cataract to treat a diabetic retinopathy, but removing the cataract may worsen the original condition.

Postoperative calamities range from infections to bleeding to corneal damage. These complications can be very serious but fortunately, are infrequent. A fairly common sequel is the clouding or hazing of the posterior capsule (the leftover skin of the grape), the so-called "second cataract." A laser beam is usually employed to clear away that area, but can, in turn, lead to other complications.

This brings up the subject of finding a good ophthalmic surgeon to do the cataract surgery once you and your optometrist deem it necessary. The best source, obviously, is the recommendation of your optometrist. He or she has probably seen many patients after the cataract extraction and has a good idea of the competence and track record of the particular ophthalmologist.

Cataract surgery has become big, big business in the United States. About 1½ million are performed every year. (Many probably are needless.) Most of them are paid for by Medicare with an annual price tag of billions of dollars. What happens when that much money is tossed around? "Cataract Centers" are born. You've undoubtedly heard and seen the advertisements for these places. Some will pick you up in a car or bus and deliver you home afterwards; some promise it won't cost you anything except co-payment, etc. in small print or quick-speak. There are two ways to look at these enterprises: (1) Because they do so many cataract surgeries, they are very proficient at it; (2) Because they must work on a large volume, the individual concern and aftercare could be less than you deserve. We think number 2 outweighs number 1 and suggest you forgo such places.

Life After an Implant

Assuming no complications and assuming that the required lens power of the IOL has been correctly calculated, your far vision will be very good and everything will seem brighter and more colorful. Remember, your aging, cataract lens was yellowish, curtailing both light and color. Many times, however, your far vision will need additional correction with glasses and, of course, you'll need help for reading. Bifocals will take care of both. (There is some experimental work being done with "bifocal" IOLs.) The increased brightness you perceive requires tinted, UV absorbing lenses to protect the retina from harmful radiation. Many intraocular lenses contain UV absorption filters, but you will certainly need sunglasses for the bright, sunny climates many seniors prefer for retirement living. (See Sunglasses.)

Other Options

There are a few instances when an implanted plastic lens cannot be used because of disease or injury. A soft contact lens will then be fitted, usually as an extended-wear option. These contacts work rather well and were used quite extensively before implants.

Prescribing and fitting glasses after cataract surgery <u>without</u> an implanted lens is difficult since very strong, thick spectacle lenses are required. Adapting to them is arduous because of the 30% enlarged image, distortions, and side vision restriction;

you'll feel clumsy when walking. If one eye is done and the other eye still has decent sight, since it is <u>impossible</u> to match the vision between the two eyes with glasses, a contact lens must be employed.

XI

The Partially Sighted

36

What Is Partially Sighted? Who Can Be Helped?

Anyone who has a sight impairment and cannot see clearly with regular glasses is considered to be partially sighted. Anyone who has a blind area in the visual field which impedes normal, spontaneous getting around, is also considered to be partially sighted.

The term "partially sighted" is rather all-encompassing because it covers a wide range of vision conditions. It can mean relatively good sight with a best corrected acuity of about 20/50 using glasses; it can mean "legal" blindness (20/200 or less); it can mean good straight ahead sight, even 20/20, but with restricted side vision; it can mean good side vision with poor straight ahead sight.

Regardless of the category, degree of sight loss, or age, improvement is usually possible. If a doctor has told you that nothing more can be done, the odds are four to one the doctor is mistaken. A very disquieting statement, but all too true. Most eye care professionals have limited knowledge about devising optical systems to make maximum use of the available sight. They will treat the disease causing the sight loss, then let the afflicted patient live with the handicap. This is quite regrettable. Ideally, there should be a joint effort by an ophthalmologist treating the disease, and an optometric low vision specialist to recoup and restore as much vision as possible.

It is difficult for a sighted person to imagine what it's like to live at the edge of blindness. Most people have the notion that all forms of blindness are what you experience when the eyes are shut. Often, it's not quite so drastic.

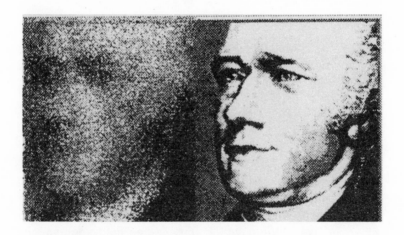

The picture on the left gives some indication of what a person might see with loss of central sight.

Legal blindness refers to a person whose corrected sight in the better eye is 20/200 or less, or when the field of view in the better eye is 20 degrees or less. With only 20/200 you'd be hard pressed to recognize faces or read anything but newspaper headlines. The restriction of a 20 degree field is almost like looking through a tube, making it awkward and difficult to walk around. (The normal panorama of view is seven to eight times larger.)

The legal definition for blindness was established in the 1930s; "corrected" means with conventional eyeglasses. The legal description is used for purposes of government assistance, income tax deductions, etc. However, it does not take into account the many new advances and aids that can assist the partially sighted person to see clearer, nor does it reveal the true ability of the individual to function out in the world.

The partially sighted person should not meekly accept this handicap until consulting an optometrist who specializes in low vision care. One of us (Herb Solomon), has been involved in low vision work for many years and is convinced that eight out of ten people can be helped.

This does not necessarily mean the improvement will reach 20/20, but it could be the difference between a grandchild's face appearing as an indistinct blur or recognizing the features; between walking hesitatingly holding a white cane or walking without assistance.

The number of totally blind people in this country is about 600,000. The number of partially sighted people is much greater, between 4,000,000 to 7,000,000 and growing. If nothing is done to keep them functioning visually, many of these people may despondently slip into the ranks of the blind.

Recent Sight Loss

For an adult, a recent and rapid loss of sight is usually accompanied by severe emotional stress. It matters little if the sight loss has been caused by disease or injury, the person's entire life is disrupted. The immediate reaction is fear—fear of not being able to carry on in the usual way, of losing a job, of being a financial burden on the family, of becoming dependent on others. Simple everyday tasks such as shaving, applying cosmetics, reading food labels, and even seeing the food on a dinner plate become very difficult and generate frustration. Is it any wonder that depression sets in? In this despondent state, the person will seek miracle cures to restore sight. ("Just make the glasses a little stronger, Doc.") The cold reality is that there's no such cure.

Going from doctor to doctor in search of a miraculous vision restoration is in itself a strong signal that you are not ready for realistic help. Unfortunately, it often takes several years of psychological soul searching to concede that you will never again see as you once did; that arduous compromises and adjustments will have to be made. Once you do come to terms with it, however, you are ready for sophisticated low vision care.

Regaining Useful Vision

Many people have a very favorable chance of regaining some useful vision. The forecast depends on the initiating cause, type and degree of vision loss, plus, and it's a big plus, the person's character and motivation. Can you be helped? Answer "yes" to at least five of the following questions and you have an excellent prognosis:

1. Do you have a strong desire to be self-sufficient, to do things without the help of others?
2. Are you willing to try new devices which may improve your sight?
3. Has your sight remained essentially the same during the past two years?
4. Can you get around fairly easily when alone in an unfamiliar place?
5. Can you recognize faces at four or more feet?
6. Can you read street signs or house numbers at five or more feet?
7. Are you light sensitive? Can you see better with less light?
8. Do you have fairly good color vision?
9. Can you read newspaper headlines or smaller print?
10. Can you read large print with a magnifying lens?

Answering "yes" to fewer than five doesn't preclude some assistance, only that the odds are not as good. If this test suggests that you can be helped, contact your family optometrist who can refer you to a low vision specialist.

When you visit the low vision specialist what can you expect? The low vision exam goes many complicated steps further than the general eye/vision examination. The goal is twofold: 1. To determine the extent of the patient's remaining vision; 2. To improve this vision with the use of special lenses, prisms, low vision aids, filters, etc., so that he/she can successfully accomplish the normal everyday tasks and/or occupation needs.

Low Vision Examination & Diagnostic Fitting

This very detailed testing regimen is usually spread over three to five visits. It gives the examiner time to understand the patient's motivational makeup, and to observe the person's visual and physical abilities under various conditions on different days. The low vision exam includes the following:

1. History.
2. Observation.
3. Evaluation of eye health.
4. Light sensitivity/color perception.
5. Visual fields.
6. Sight using optical (lenses, telescopes, microscopes) and non-optical aids.

The doctor will request background information which can be helpful. To save time and assure accuracy of this information, most offices will mail a questionnaire to be filled out at your leisure at home. (See a typical form on page 241.)

CASE HISTORY: With the completed questionnaire in hand, the history of the condition as well as your expectations and readiness to accept low vision aids will be explored at greater length. What's most important for you—distance vision, reading, driving an automobile, sewing, watching TV? What compromises are you willing to make?

OBSERVATION: A great deal of information can be obtained by carefully watching the patient. What to look for? How the person walks into the room avoiding obstacles gives a good indication of side vision. The person's head may be held in an unusual position to compensate for a blind area in the field of vision or because of an unusual light sensitivity; the direction of gaze may be off-center to shun a blind spot. These and other observed facts have to be considered before low vision aids can be successfully prescribed.

EVALUATION OF EYE HEALTH: If the sight loss is caused by a disease condition, it's important to differentiate between a stable ailment and one that is progressing in severity. For example, if uncontrolled glaucoma, diabetes or circulatory problems exist, only temporary visual aids will be considered until the condition stabilizes. On the other hand, since most inherited conditions that stem from a dominant genetic trait (nystagmus, retinitis pigmentosa, aniridia, etc.) conform to a reasonably predictable pattern, more permanent aids can be prescribed.

SIGHT ASSESSMENT: How much can you naturally see? This is more difficult to determine than it sounds. Because the visual capability of the partially sighted person is affected by lighting, contrast, color, and even fatigue, it takes a longer time to evaluate. It is also vital to document these variations in designing the proper low vision aids.

VISUAL FIELDS: More often than not, there is some loss of side vision or "blank" areas in the field of view. The initial visual field test will record the loss and by repeating the test at intervals of weeks or months, it will accurately track any changes that may have occurred.

DIAGNOSTIC FITTING: Think of this as a trial run to test the patient with different optical aids, such as magnifiers, telescopes, microscopes, prisms, etc. in order to determine the sight improvement that is possible. This always takes several office visits.

Since better sight in the office setting does not necessarily translate to useful sight in the real world, don't be surprised if some of the testing is done out of doors. Doing this also affords the opportunity to demonstrate if tints and/or filters are useful.

By the time all these tests and office visits are concluded, both the doctor and the patient will have a very good idea of how much improvement is possible.

Herbert Solomon, O.D., F.A.A.O.

6201 N. California
Chicago, Illinois 60659

(312) 743-0100

Please fill out as completely as possible and bring at first visit.

Name_____ Birthdate_____

Address_____City_____Zip_____

Telephone_____Occupation_____

Name of relative or friend to contact_____Telephone_____

Name of your optometrist_____Telephone_____

Name of your ophthalmologist_____Telephone_____

Name of general physician/internist_____Telephone_____

EYE HEALTH INFORMATION:

When did you first notice sight loss_____

Diagnosis of your eye condition_____

Eye surgery or laser treatment_____

   When_____Which eye_____

Eye medication_____

GENERAL HEALTH INFORMATION

List health problems_____

List drugs/medications_____

List all optical aids used (i.e., eyeglasses, magnifiers, etc.)_____

_____

List all non-optical aids (i.e., special lights, large print books, etc.)_____

_____

37

The Young Visually Impaired

THE CHILD: Discovering that your child has a serious visual problem bordering on blindness is a devastating experience. Not counting eye injuries, such problems are usually brought on by congenital conditions or hereditary defects. The congenital cases are frequently caused by a viral infection or the use of drugs during pregnancy. We are not only referring to illicit drugs, but even medication legally prescribed by physicians.

The most common conditions causing sight impairment in children are: Albinism (lack of pigment), scarring of the cornea, nystagmus (rapid, oscillating eye movements), amblyopia, degenerative myopia, and injuries.

Can this child lead a reasonably normal life? Is regular schooling possible? The answer to each question is a qualified "yes." If the child has a stable, congenital condition, he or she can be helped rather easily to see better and have a fairly normal life. Children have a knack for adjusting to new situations, and quickly learn to use optical aids. They will even adopt ways of seeing which may seem strange to you. For instance, it is not unusual for a child with poor distant sight to be able to read small print held a few inches away. The reason is the large amount of focusing power available to the young eye. By taking advantage of it, the child may get along quite well in school, using only telescopic spectacles to see the chalkboard.

Schools across the country handle the partially sighted child in different ways. Some will lump them all together in classes for the visually handicapped; others will base the separation on the degree of attainable functional vision. The ideal program places the child in the regular classroom so that both the sighted and partially sighted can associate together. With additional help from resource teachers and special resource material, it will usually be possible for the child to attend regular classes and follow the same curriculum. We urge each school district to obtain the services of an optometric low vision specialist to evaluate each child individually.

In the classroom, the child's seating must be carefully chosen. It is not just a matter of being close to the chalkboard, though that may be necessary. The partially sighted child must be in a seat which is compatible with his individual lighting requirements. Some require strong illumination, others need low levels. For example, an albino child may have to be shielded from sunlight streaming through the window, and use tinted lenses, side shields, or even a visor to screen overhead light. Another child may need a good desk lamp to light the reading material. Reflections from shiny surfaces, only mildly annoying to a normal child, can be a serious visual irritant.

Some of these youngsters will require writing guides, special pencils and heavily lined notebook paper. Since it usually takes a little longer to complete assignments, the teachers should provide extra time. Participation in most school activities can be encouraged, but if the child has only one functional eye, body contact sports are to be avoided.

If you keep in mind that good sight is only one part of the complex system we call vision you will realize that while it's very important, correcting the sight is not enough. We advocate that the child be given visual therapy for better eye movements, hand eye coordination, establish patterns for the two eyes to work together, etc. Some of this therapy can be done in the school, closely supervised by the teacher and monitored by the optometrist.

So far we've been discussing the school-age child. What about the younger child? Depending on the child's ability to understand their use, optical aids for sight improvement can be prescribed. The optometrist will guide the parents in setting up a visual development program for the child. Just as you must walk to develop the leg muscles, the eye must be stimulated to learn to see. If the problem is juvenile cataracts, for example, the cataracts must be removed at the earliest possible time so that the system can learn to see. After a successful operation glasses or contact lenses can improve the sight dramatically.

Contact lenses can, and are, prescribed for very young children. Soft lenses are infinitely safer. The contacts have to be inserted and removed by an adult, but this is one of the few genuine uses for extended-wear lenses. Other situations which lend themselves beautifully to contacts are cases of scarred or irregular corneas, degenerative myopia, and when very strong corrections are needed.

Contact lenses are only one example of novel ways to enable your child to see. We find that some parents are reluctant to allow the fitting of unusual devices because of some vague feeling that it may "use up" the child's vision. This myth belongs in the same wastebasket as the belief that you can "use up" your brain by learning or remembering too much. A few parents veto strange looking optical aids because it makes the child look different from other children. We can sympathize with this feeling, but depriving the child of vision is too much of a penalty to pay. Marvelous things are possible when you open your mind and allow your child to see.

TEENAGER; YOUNG ADULT: The education of the partially sighted teenager should be geared to the vocational possibilities that will be open to him or her. It's a good idea to get advice from the optometrist, an ophthalmologist, educator, vocational guidance counselor, etc. Keep in mind that visually handicapped people are often met with the same prejudices in obtaining employment as totally blind people.

Students with moderate visual handicaps, which we can define by rule of thumb as poor distance vision but adequate near vision, usually have little difficulty completing high school. As with normal sighted students, success with schoolwork as well as the ability to enter college, depends on intelligence, motivation, interest, and aptitudes. If the near vision is good enough to read textbook print, these students, with additional help as needed from special resource teachers, can attend regular classes. (Of course, distance vision will have to be corrected with telescopic aids.) The optometrist should work closely with the teachers to determine if the visual needs are being met. For example, if near seeing becomes troublesome in the upper grades, reading glasses may be needed.

There is one visual area which is usually very blurry for the partially sighted and often neglected—the intermediate range from about ten inches to three feet. This is the working range for such things as typing, computer pursuit, laboratory experiments in chemistry and physics, and shop work. If at all practical, the student may try to "poke his nose" to within a few inches to see the work, otherwise he will just give up and avoid the task. The alert low vision specialist will prescribe special visual aids such as near telescopes, hand magnifiers and adjustable reading stands to cope with these situations. When this is done, a new dimension is opened for the student.

It is much easier to plan the educational and vocational future for the teenager with a stable, moderate, visual handicap. The stable condition assures fewer changes of low vision aids, and the moderate condition does not severely limit the choice of job opportunities. The only real limitation would be work requiring critical distance seeing, i.e., driving a bus, operating a crane etc. On the other hand, many blue-collar and most white-collar jobs are quite suitable. Searching through newspaper want-ads reveals that about 80% of the listed jobs can be managed successfully (provided hiring prejudices are overcome).

If the visual impairment is severe or rapidly worsening, finishing high school and college becomes an arduous task. We have to resort to stronger, hence more limiting visual aids (large print books, projection devices) and obtain the services of trained readers. Besides the elimination of jobs requiring critical distance seeing when thinking about a vocation, there is the limitation imposed by how much vision improvement is possible at near. Most blue-collar and many white-collar jobs have to be passed up, but some can be handled. For instance, becoming a bank teller would be impractical, but becoming a credit analyst in that same bank would be appropriate.

When the person is no longer able to keep up visually with the printed work assignments, or if the prognosis is for nearly total blindness, braille should be mastered and preparations made for jobs relying on hearing and touch. Young people have little difficulty becoming proficient in braille and learn to utilize it concurrently with their visual aids.

38

The Partially Sighted
as a Driver

Incredible as it sounds, it's possible to be legally blind and
receive a driver's license (lawfully) in more that half the
states. It isn't done with sleight of hand, but with a
telescopic viewing system and/or telescopic glasses. Some
states will grant a license if you can demonstrate 20/70 sight;
some require 20/50 or 20/40. However, merely being able to
see 20/70, 20/40, or even 20/20, does not make someone a safe
driver. There are visual and mobility skills which are just as
indispensable as sight. Before undertaking the lengthy process
leading to obtaining a driver's license for a partially sighted
person, the following is required:

1. A stable vision condition which will not change in the
    near future.
2. Adequate color vision to clearly distinguish red from
    green traffic signals.
3. Unrestricted eye movements and the ability to look
    quickly from one object to another.

4. Normal and unrestricted head movements.
5. A field of view encompassing about 130 degrees with each eye, and no significant blind or missing areas.

To understand the significance of a wide field of view when driving, imagine your car windows fogged up except for one small, clear area directly ahead of you. No matter how well you can see through that clear spot, it obviously would be very dangerous to drive. Normal peripheral vision extends about 90 degrees outward from each eye; less than 70 degrees is not acceptable. Since only some states test the field of vision, it's up to the optometrist to determine if the partially sighted person meets the minimum requirements.

The preferred way to improve sight for driving is with the telescopic viewing system (contact lenses plus glasses). Once you have adapted to this setup, you should be able to drive fairly normally. The hitch for many partially sighted persons is that this system only works well with moderate sight losses. For those needing greater sight improvements we resort to wide angle, bioptic telescopes. It takes patience, practice, and time (two to four months) to reach the point where you can use these glasses "automatically." You have to adjust to such things as objects popping in and out of the field of view with your eye movements. Before allowing you to take the driving test, the low vision specialist will work closely with the driving instructor to make sure of your proficiency under traffic conditions.

At the present time, Dr. Solomon has patients who have obtained driver's licenses and are safely handling automobiles while wearing sophisticated telescopic aids and systems.

For many partially sighted persons, driving an auto is at the bottom of their list of priorities. But, if it's important, help may be a close as your low vision specialist.

39

Optical/Non-Optical Aids

Very often the partially-sighted person is left on his own to find a better way to see. He may drift into a department store and try the use of a hand magni fier; a well-meaning friend or relative may present him with one as a gift. Though the basic idea is sound and he may derive some benefits from the magnifier, they will be limited because: (a) the magnifiers generally available on the retail market are of low power; (b) he may not know how to use it effectively; (c) it will only be useful for a particular task; or (d) if it doesn't work, he will reject all magnifiers.

Normally, the human eye can see across a wide range of distances. For the partially-sighted person this ability is sharply curtailed. Consequently, a number of different aids are needed for seeing at different distances. It all depends on the amount of visual loss, what precisely needs to be seen and how far away it is.

Let's illustrate this concept with Mrs. L., a sixty-year-old woman with only 10% vision left after retinal degeneration. For television and movies she uses tiny telescopes fused to her glasses. For cooking and doing housework within a distance of a few feet, she uses near bioptic telescopes and a hand magnifier. Last, for reading or close detail work, she uses very strong reading glasses with intense lighting. To the sighted person, this multiplicity of aids might seem cumbersome and complicated. For Mrs. L., blind for all practical purposes without them, they represent access to the sighted world and she is delighted. Of course, not all partially-sighted patients require the same help Mrs. L. has been given. The point is, however, the various visual needs of the individual must be evaluated and satisfied, if possible.

The underlying theory for improving sight is to make the object larger and bolder, hence easier to recognize. How can this be accomplished? The simplest way is to actually enlarge the size of the object. In this category are non-optical aids such as large print books, magazines, and newspapers; large numbers on telephone dials; large eyes in needles, etc. It is impractical to rely entirely on this solution; the material is often not available.

Another way to enlarge what you want to see is by relative size magnification. This simply means that the closer you get to an object, the larger it appears. For instance, newspaper print which the partially-sighted person cannot read at sixteen inches, might well be legible at eight inches because it is relatively twice as large; at four inches it appears four times as large. The print is not actually any larger, but by bringing it closer, the image on the retina is enlarged. That leaves only one complication—the eye must be able to focus at a very close distance. Partially-sighted children have little problem since at their age they have great focusing ability. The older person is not as fortunate because focusing ability decreases with age. The optometrist overcomes this by prescribing optical aids to make things clear at the very close viewing distance. It can be done with special microscopic glasses, magnifiers, or loupes attached to glasses.

That takes care of near seeing, but what about looking at television or movies? The only solution is a device which has the ability to enlarge distant objects, namely, a telescope. Some partially-sighted persons who require very high magnification in order to see, actually watch television through binoculars (two telescopes side by side). As you can imagine, it becomes very fatiguing and annoying to hold them still; slight movements cause the image to waver and jump.

A much more convenient method is to use telescopic clip-ons over spectacles. Though the view through them is rather narrow, it's sufficiently wide to see a TV screen at about ten feet. However, the telescopic clip-ons are useless for walking around.

The most functional and convenient system which does permit walking, is a tiny telescope permanently attached to the upper part of the spectacles. Compact and light in weight, it has enough power and an adequate field of view to be useful for extended periods of time. This design is called a bioptic telescope and works like an upside-down bifocal. For regular seeing and walking, the person looks through the lower part of the spectacle lenses; for a magnified, clearer view of TV, faces, street signs, etc., he lowers his head slightly to look through the telescope. The usefulness of bioptics can be enhanced by adding lens "caps" which are made for looking at objects closer than three feet. It is also possible to design bioptics to see with both eyes. More recently, bioptic telescopes with a built-in, adjustable "zoom" attachment permits easier focusing of nearby objects. When a wider field of view is desired, the "honey bee" type of bioptic telescope has some advantages. It takes its name from the eye of a bee because of its unusual appearance. Three small telescopes are fused side by side on the upper portion of the glasses.

Modern technology has made it possible to make the telescopes very tiny, but the principal goes back to Galileo who discovered that two lenses of opposite power, separated by a given distance, can enlarge an image. A new and interesting way to approach this is by using a contact lens combined with strong glasses, on the eye. While the possible magnification is limited, it works wonderfully for some people. The fitting of such an arrangement requires critical planning and execution. Sometimes it is combined with bioptic telescopes in the glasses for greater benefits. Dr. Solomon has done pioneering work in this field with considerable success.

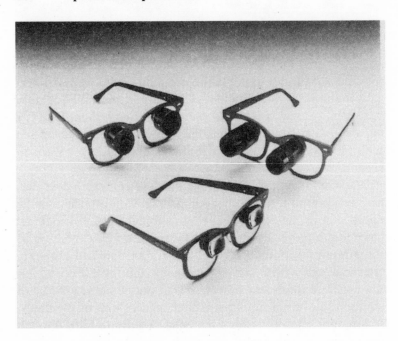

Some examples of bioptic telescopic glasses.

Up to now, we have discussed the help available for the partially sighted person with poor central vision, but good peripheral vision. Now let's discuss that segment of the low vision population that has fairly good central vision but very limited side vision. There are two notable eye diseases responsible for this, retinitis pigmentosa and glaucoma. These people require systems to improve their side vision and ability to get around by themselves.

Although designing these systems is a difficult task, it can be done in three ways:

1. Using prisms cemented to the spectacle lens. Objects in the blind, peripheral areas are displaced inward where they can be seen.

2. With small mirrors attached to the frame of the glasses. You may have seen this idea used by bicycle riders to see behind them. Glancing into an appropriately angled mirror will bring the missing side area into view.

3. By Minification. Reducing the size of things will now bring more of the world into the constricted central

seeing area. If this concept is difficult to understand, you're probably familiar with your car's right-side mirror that gives a wide panorama because of minification. Another example would be the tiny, minifying "peep-hole" lens that allows a wide view of objects on the other side of a door

In practice, a small bioptic miniscope with your prescription is fused into the upper part of your regular glasses. By simply raising your gaze, a wider field can be seen.

Another, more recent development is the amorphic lens. The idea originated with the wide-screen movies popular several decades ago. If you recall, the side view is expanded, but the height remains the same. This concept has been adapted and is available for low vision patients.

A more novel approach combines the use of contact lenses and high-power spectacles for expanding the field of vision.

About 25% of the people with restricted side vision can be helped. Although most people using these special lens systems still require a cane to get around safely, some can discard the cane and function with one of the minifying systems.

There is a great variety of non-optical aids available for the low vision patient. With these, everyday tasks in the home, out of doors, in the workplace and recreational activities can be easier to perform and even fun.

Included are aids for education/teaching, reading, writing, health care, household, recreation, watches, clocks and timers, calculators, games, communication, light protection shields, music, large print books and publications, illumination, mobility, tools, measuring, computers, and more.

Catalogs containing a complete list of products can be obtained by telephoning or writing to:

1. American Foundation for the Blind
   100 Enterprise Place
   Dover, DE 19903-7044
2. American Library Association
   50 East Huron Street
   Chicago, IL 60611
3. American Printing House for the Blind
   1839 Frankfort Avenue
   Louisville, KY

4. Braille Institute of America
   741 Vermont Avenue
   Los Angeles, CA
5. Independent Living Aids, Inc.
   27 East Mall
   Plainview, NY 11803
6. Large Print Clearing House
   P.O. Box 624
   Colville, WA 99114
   Telephone (509) 732-4842
7. Library of Congress
   Division for the Blind and Physically Handicapped
   Washington, DC
8. The Lighthouse
   3602 Northern Boulevard
   Long Island City, NY 11101
   Telephone (718) 937-6959
9. L S and S Group, Inc.
   P.O. Box 673
   Northbrook, IL 60065
   Telephone (1-800) 468-4789
10. New York Association for the
    Blind
    111 East 59th Street
    New York, NY 10022
    Telephone (212) 355-2200
11. Science Products
    Box 888
    Southeastern, PA 19399
12. Independent Living Aids, Inc.
    27 East Mall
    Plainview, New York 11803

Guide to Optical Aids for the Partially Sighted

Type of Aid	How Used	When Used	Comments
I. Telescopes A. Binoculars 1. Handheld	One or both eyes. Adjustable focus.	For distance magnification Distance viewing, 5 feet or more. TV, sports, faces, street signs, etc.	Available in various magnifications. Field size depends on lens size and power. Wide angle available
	One eye only.	Near viewing. For near work and intermediate distances. Writing, reading labels on shelves, etc.	Limited to tasks of short duration. Difficult to use if hands unsteady. Small field of view.
2. Ready-made binoculars in eyeglass frame	One or both eyes.	For distance viewing. TV, movies, theatre, sports, etc.	Available in up to 3X magnification only. Relatively inexpensive. Can't be used if lens presecription required. Small field of view.
3. Headband type	Fits on head. Can be worn over glasses or swung out of way.	Near viewing, 3–10 inches. Useful for light-sensitive eyes. Best if sight about equal in both eyes.	Fairly wide field, 2–4 inches, depending on power. Good stereoscopic effect. Frees use of hands.

Guide to Optical Aids for the Partially Sighted (cont'd)

Type of Aid	How Used	When Used	Comments
4. Bioptics	One or both eyes. Telescopes fused to upper part of glasses. Patient's Rx in system.	Distance viewing as walking, driving. When normal and magnified seeing is needed. School, travel, etc.	Up to 6X magnification at distance. Can be worn at all times. Easy to use. Rx changes can be made. Expensive. Wide angle available. Must be accurately centered.
	One eye only. Lens attachments for near and intermediate, or adjustable.	Intermediate and near viewing.. Typing, music, etc.	
5. Near telescopes	Telescopes fused to lower part of glasses and angled to permit use of both eyes. Patient's Rx in upper part.	When reading distances of 5–40 inches needed. Also typing, cooking, etc.	Up to 8X magnification. Relatively small field of view. Careful adjustment essential. Least amount of distortion.
B. Monoculars (Handheld, attachable, fused)	One eye only. Can be clipped onto glasses, adjustable focus,	Distance viewing, TV, school, sports, etc.	Attachable, available up to 3X magnification, fused up to 4X, handheld up to 10X. Inexpensive. Not for walking.

Guide to Optical Aids for the Partially Sighted (cont'd)

Type of Aid	How Used	When Used	Comments
II. Magnifiers			
A. Monocular			
1. Clip-ons	Attached to temple or frame front. Either eye can be used. Can be flipped out of way.	Near viewing, 1½–40 inches. When strong near glasses needed but bifocal not practical. Best as a temporary aid when vision is changing.	Inexpensive and lightweight. Available with side shields for persons bothered by scattered light. Frees hands to hold reading material.
B. Binocular			
1. Clip-ons	Attached to regular glasses. Available as flip-up.	Near viewing from 4–40 inches.	Inexpensive.
C. Spectacles	Worn in ordinary eyeglass frame as bifocal, ½ eye or full reading glasses.	When large field is needed. Strong powers for seeing as close as ½ inch from eye available. Two eyes can be used as close as 4 inches.	Frees hands to hold reading material. Cosmetically acceptable. Can be tinted for light sensitive persons. Not for use with small visual fields as in advanced glaucoma. Relatively inexpensive except in very strong powers.
D. Handheld (Available with handles, pocket size, folding type, illuminating attachments. Glass or plastic)	Best magnification at set distance. Can be used over bifocals. Available from 1X to 17X. Powers over 5X should be held close to eyes for widest field. Can be suspended from neck to free hands.	For reading and certain occupations where longer reading needed. Checking dials, meters, price tags, invoice numbers. For sewing, knitting, reading food labels, cooking directions, etc.	Inexpensive. Useful when sensitive about appearance of other aids. Difficult to use with unsteady hands. Holding magnifiers close to eyes enlarges field of view.

Guide to Optical Aids for the Partially Sighted (cont'd)

Type of Aid	How Used	When Used	Comments
E. Stand			
1. Fixed-focus	Lens placed over material. Rests on a stand. Patient must use bifocal or have focusing ability.	For greater reading distances. For patient who cannot hold hand magnifier steady.	Magnification from 1X–20X possible. Easy to use.
2. Adjustable focus	Must be used close to eye with attachable illumination. No bifocal needed.	When patient has very poor sight and little or no focusing ability.	Very strong powers available. Very limited field of view.
III. Projection magnifiers	Enlarges reading material by projecting it on a screen. Either optical or electronic with TV screen.	When sight is very limited. Up to 40X magnification possible. Can be used for writing. Has typewriter attachment.	Electronic magnifier is not easily portable. Newer devices have good quality picture with variable illumination. Can be used in comfortable sitting position.

Guide to Non-Optical Aids for the Partially Sighted

Type of Aid	How It Is Used	Where Obtainable
A. Writing aids		
1. Bold lined paper	Easier to write along a straight line. Helps keep place. Available for all grades of school and for letter writing	American Printing House for the Blind
2. Check writing guide	For easier location of name, amount and signature on checks. Cut to order.	American Foundation for the Blind
3. Porous tip pens	These pens write with darker, bolder lines. Easier to read your own writing. Come in many thicknesses and color.	Most stationery, variety and department stores
4. Letter writing guide	For proper spacing of sentences and to write in a straight line.	American Foundation for the Blind
B. Reading, typing stands and racks		
1. Adjustable table reading stand	Convenient holder for any size book. Adjustable to many angles.	New York Association for the Blind
2. Desk top reading stand clips stand clips	Holds any width book, portable and can be used in classroom.	American Printing House for the Blind
3. Adjustable reading stands	The height, angle, distance, and position of reading material can be easily controlled. Also useful for music and typing.	Stationery stores

259

Guide to Non-Optical Aids for the Partially Sighted (cont'd)

Type of Aid	How It Is Used	Where Obtainable
4. Attachable reading stands	Can be clamped to table tops, desks. Fully adjustable.	American Printing House for the Blind
5. Coore reading stand	For 6–12 inch distances. Holds large books, music, typing material.	American Printing House for the Blind
6. Shafer reading stand	Floor model adjustable for standing or sitting at any angle.	American Printing House for the Blind
C. Light shields 1. Visors	Attached to head. Protects from glare and overhead light.	Stationery, department stores
2. Visorette	As above, but attached to glasses.	New York Association for the Blind
3. Side shields	Protects from glare, dust, dirt. Fastens sides of glasses. Opaque or tinted.	Optical houses
4. Wrap around clip-on clip-on sun–	Plastic lenses clipped on the inside of frames for glare protection.	Optical houses
5. Noir sun glasses	Only known plastic lens which filters out infra-red rays. Two densities allow either 7% or 17% light to enter eye. Worn over glasses. Useful after cataract surgery.	Optical houses

Guide to Non-Optical Aids for the Partially Sighted (cont'd)

Type of Aid	How It Is Used	Where Obtainable
D. Aids for music		
1. Large type music staff paper	For hand transcribing music.	American Printing House for the Blind
2. Notation-draft board	Includes notes and material to construct music phrases, etc. For people with very limited sight.	American Printing House for the Blind
3. Music racks	Designed for upright piano. Adjustable to many distances and angles.	American Printing House for the Blind
E. Large print books and publications	Wide range of material available. Fiction, non-fiction, technical, religious, etc.	Keith Jennison Books American Printing House for the Blind Large Print Publications American Bible Society
F. Dictionaries	Large print for school, home, etc.	Books, Inc. Stanwix House
G. Large print newspapers	Enlarged print *New York Times* published weekly.	*New York Times*
H. Large telephone dials	Large numbers for easier dialing.	Telephone Company New York Association for the Blind
I. Playing cards	Standard cards with enlarged numbers	New York Association for the Blind

Guide to Non-Optical Aids for the Partially Sighted (cont'd)

Type of Aid	How It Is Used	Where Obtainable
J. Special illumination		
1. Lamps	Adjustable gooseneck and spring arm to concentrate light where needed.	Lamp stores, stationers
2. High intensity lamps	Strong, small concentrated light such as Tensor, Luxo, Lightolier, etc.	Lamp stores, stationers

XII

Eye Diseases, Injuries, Disorders

40

Emergencies

Emergency information falls into two categories: Knowing what constitutes a medical crisis that requires prompt attention, and then knowing what to do to minimize the damage.

Blow to the Eye

Being hit in the eye is the most common potentially serious type of injury to the eye. While a "black eye" is often a topic for levity, it can be a grave situation even leading to blindness. Any severe blow should be examined either by your eye doctor or someone in a hospital emergency room. The pain and swelling can be moderated with a cold compress. The list of possible damage from a blow includes: fractured orbital bones, torn iris muscles, displaced crystalline lens, retinal detachment, internal bleeding, and muscle entrapment.

Fortunately, in many cases, the soft eye is protected by the bony orbit (socket) and eyebrow ridge. When this area takes the brunt of the blow, the bleeding will be limited to underneath the skin around the eye and produce the classic black eye. Without further complications, the blood will be absorbed in about a week. The skin may also be cut, and is treated as any cut.

If the emergency room personnel assure you that it's only a black eye, they will also advise that you see your eye doctor for follow-up care. Any ache or restricted eye movements should be gone in a day or two. If not, be certain to visit your eye doctor. Even if everything looks and feels normal in a week, you are not necessarily home free. There is the possibility of a retinal tear or secondary glaucoma happening weeks or even years later.

Foreign Object or Particle in the Eye

Everyone gets something in the eye from time to time. A piece of dust, eyelash, or wool fuzz will cause liberal tearing and discomfort. If the tearing does not wash the particle away, try to gently remove it with the edge of a tissue or cotton swab. If this doesn't work and the eye is painful and very light sensitive, get professional help.

Your activity just before you felt something in your eye is very important. If you were hammering, doing sanding, cutting tree branches, drilling through metal, etc., the probability is higher that the particle has penetrated the surface of the cornea or eye and is firmly embedded. It's even possible that the particle has perforated the outer shell of the eye and is lodged somewhere inside. These injuries require urgent professional evaluation, removal of the offending particle and follow-up care. Embedded plant material can cause a secondary infection and reaction; a metal particle may leave a rust ring on the cornea.

Chemical Burns

Regardless of whether the chemical is an acid or alkali, IMMEDIATELY flood the eye with water holding the lids open as wide as possible for a MINIMUM of 30 minutes. To understand the importance of not wasting time, an alkali chemical such as ammonia, lye, or fireworks powder in strong concentration can penetrate the eye in only 15 seconds. Acid chemicals are slightly less dangerous because the cornea can somewhat neutralize acids. A water drinking fountain is excellent because it's easy to keep your head in the correct position. Otherwise, tilt your face under a faucet and keep the water running continuously. After this is done, get to an eye doctor or emergency room.

It would be wise to memorize the previous paragraph. If it happens to you, there won't be time to look up the information.

Thermal Burns

If the eye and/or lids are burned by fire or a hot liquid, hold a cool, wet compress to the eye and get immediate medical attention.

Radiation (Sunlight, welding, sunlamp, intense heat) Burns

A corneal burn caused by ultraviolet radiation from a sunlamp or welding is insidious because you won't feel much until 8 to 10 hours after the event. Chances are you'll be awakened from sleep by the intense pain. Contact your eye doctor for necessary treatment, although it's generally self healing. If there are no complications, the injury to the cornea will resolve in about 36 hours. (Most people wear appropriate protective goggles when facing a sunlamp, but may foolishly read a book without the goggles and have the UV reflect off the pages.)

A "flash" burn from an intense heat (infrared) source is felt right away and could have more serious consequences depending on the severity.

Sudden Loss of Sight

Sudden, painless loss of sight in one eye is caused by a blocked central retinal artery or vein. There is little time to wait to seek treatment, although even with treatment the prospect of regaining full sight is poor. Irreparable damage to retinal tissue can occur in an hour. If you lose sight in only part of the visual field it means that a branch artery or vein is blocked and the outlook for at least partial recovery is better.

You can experience similar sight-loss symptoms from a temporary blockage or blood vessel spasm which will last from a couple of minutes to about 15 minutes. Best advice: Set out for emergency treatment. If the sight returns while you're en route, you can wait to report it to your optometrist/ophthalmologist and physician. Persons with circulatory problems are most susceptible for this occurrence.

Flashing or Sparkling Lights

This could be an emergency if it signals a retinal detachment. With a detachment you will also see something that looks like a greyish, descending veil or spider web. Flashing or sparkling lights can also precede a migraine headache, and accompany a blood vessel/circulation problem. If you are an older person and see occasional flashes to the extreme side, mostly at night, it's probably caused by tugging of the vitreous at its attachment point to the retina. This is rarely an emergency but it should be reported to your optometrist for evaluation.

Descending Veil or Spider Web

See previous.

Insect Stings, Allergic Reactions

An insect sting on the lids is only an emergency if you are hyper-allergic and have a history of severe reactions. People who are, usually know it. Mostly it will cause smarting, burning and some swelling. If the stinger is still set in the skin, flick it out with your fingers. Don't try to grasp it or it may only pump more venom into the site. A cold cloth or ice pack should help relieve the symptoms.

Blood-red Eye

You may wake up some morning, look into the mirror and find, to your alarm, a bright red eye staring back at you. Or someone may call your attention to it during the day. When there are no other symptoms of disease (pain, for instance), this is simply a hemorrhage of a tiny conjunctival blood vessel. The appearance is very dramatic because the overlying tissue is transparent and the blood is visible. Usually, the cause is some strain or pressure such as lifting a heavy weight or strenuous coughing or sneezing (even during sleep.) High blood pressure may also be the culprit or contributor. Cool compresses several times a day for the first 2 days, then warm compresses to facilitate the absorption, is helpful. To be on the safe side, have your eye doctor take a look at it.

Painful, Red Eye

A sore, red eye with light sensitivity, blurred vision and a tiny, constricted pupil usually signals iritis. This is an inflammation of the iris, the colored part of the eye. The cause could be a systemic illness or physical insult to the eye. While this is not an extreme emergency, you should get early treatment.

If the painful, red eye develops very rapidly (less than an hour) and is accompanied by nausea, headache, vision reduction and an enlarged, dilated pupil it could well be an acute glaucoma attack. This is an unusual condition; most glaucomas are slow-developing without pain. However, if you're the 1 in about 25,000 people, get professional attention as quickly as possible to avoid permanent sight loss.

Minimizing the Risk

Many of these emergencies can be avoided by simply using common sense. Wear protective goggles when you are working with dangerous chemicals, including handling automobile batteries. Carpentry should never be undertaken without safety glasses. Also wear them around high speed machinery, when chipping paint, tinkering underneath an auto, etc.

Keep a list of phone numbers of your doctors in a handy place.

41

External Parts

I. LIDS

1. Blepharitis: Inflammation of the lid margin with redness and swelling. It may be associated with allergies and dandruff scales. In the mild form there is a crusting of the lash bases. Some lashes fall out, but grow back. Severe blepharitis (ulcerative) affects the lash follicles; there is a permanent loss of lashes with distortion of the lid margin.

2. External hordeolum or sty: Infection of a hair follicle (similar to a boil). It begins with a general swelling and pain of the lid, then localizes into a red area with a yellowish center at the lid margin. Breaks open to discharge pus and heals readily.

3. Chalazion: Chronic, sometimes inflammatory enlargement of one of the lid glands. Appears as a bump or swelling which slowly increases in size. There is usually no pain.

4. Internal hordeolum or sty: Infection of a gland on the underside of the lid.

5. Ptosis: Drooping of the upper lid. It may be a congenital condition due to a paralysis of the lid muscles or a neurological disorder. Mostly, however, it is seen in older people when there is a loss of muscle tone.

6. Entropion: The margin of the lid turns inward causing the lashes to rub and irritate the cornea. Occurs most often in older people or following an injury or a burn.

7. Ectropion: The margin of the lid turns outward causing excessive tearing as well as itching and burning of the exposed inner lid. Occurs usually in older people from loss of muscle tone.

8. Cysts and Tumors:

(a) *Xanthelasma:* Flat, yellowish, fatty growth on the surface of the lids, especially near the inner corner. It causes no problem unless there are many large ones which are cosmetically unacceptable.

(b) *Cyst of gland of Moll:* Small, transparent, watery cyst at the lid margin.

(c) *Nevus:* Benign tumor which may be pigmented. It is frequently present from birth, but goes unnoticed until it begins to enlarge later in life. In only very rare cases does it become malignant.

(d) *Malignant tumors:* Can involve any of the cell layers of the lids. The majority occur on the lower lid.

9. Trachoma: A viral infection of the inside lid. It gives a granular, cobblestone appearance. It is uncommon in the U.S., but is a major cause of blindness in some parts of the world.

10. Trichiasis: One or more lashes grow inward and cause irritation by rubbing the cornea.

11. Dacryocystitis: Infection of the tear drainage sac located near the inner corner of the eye. Mild cases exhibit some redness and slight swelling. Severe cases cause pain and obvious swelling.

II. CONJUNCTIVA

Thin transparent membrane covering the inner surface of the lid and the surface (white) of the eye.

1. Conjunctivitis: The common "red eye" or "pink eye."

(a) *Allergic:* The main symptom is itching accompanied by redness. In some cases the inside surface of the upper lid becomes involved with cobblestone-shaped elevations and a thick secretion.

(b) *Infectious (bacterial):* The symptoms are itching, tearing, sensitivity to light, and a gritty sensation. The condition can be acute or drag on as a mild, chronic infection. The lids may be stuck together from the discharge, especially when awakening in the morning.

(c) *Infectious (viral):* The symptoms are similar to the bacterial type but frequently the cornea becomes involved with serious consequences.

2. Hemorrhage: A spontaneous hemorrhage can occur on the white of the eye giving a bright, blood-red appearance. Sometimes it is caused by coughing, sneezing, or rubbing the eyes too hard.

3. Pinguecula: A small, yellowish elevation on the white of the eye, usually on the nasal side. It becomes more noticeable with age, but is harmless.

4. Pterygium: A triangular shaped elevated, vascular tissue on the white of the eye. It is harmless unless it grows across the cornea and blocks sight.

III. CORNEA

The clear cover in front of the colored part of the eye.

1. Arcus senilis: A partial or complete grey or whitish ring near the edge of the cornea. While very common with aging, it can indicate an elevated cholesterol level.

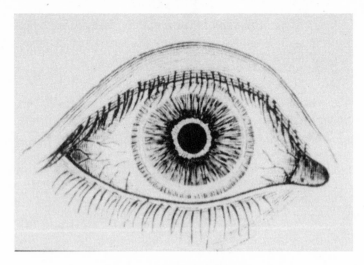

Arcus senilis

2. *Keratitis:* An inflammation of the cornea.

(a) *Superficial:* The infection starts on the surface from an outside source. Depending on the infecting agent, various ulcerations can occur leaving opaque scars after healing.

(b) *Deep:* Transmitted via the blood stream and usually confined to inner layers. The most common type is caused by congenital syphilis and will show up in children and teenagers.

3. *Keratoconus:* The central area of the cornea becomes thin and bulges forward into a conical shape. Vision is always affected.

4. *Abrasion:* A breakdown of the surface layer of the cornea accompanied by pain, tearing, and light sensitivity. Injury or contact lens wear are usually the causes.

5. *Vascularization:* The blood vessels invade the cornea (which is devoid of any vessels). It can be caused by disease, inflammation, or injury.

6. *Ulceration:* Erosion of the corneal surface caused by bacteria, fungus, or virus. It always causes scarring and in extreme cases may perforate through the entire cornea.

IV. SCLERA

The tough, white outer layer of the eyeball.

1. *Episcleritis:* Inflammation of the loose connective tissue of the sclera. It looks very much like conjunctivitis, except that it is usually restricted to a small area, and is a deep red or purple color.

2. *Staphyloma:* A small pigmented bulge in the white of the eye caused by a thinning of the sclera.

42

Internal Parts

I. IRIS

A thin, pigmented membrane lying in front of the lens. The pupil is the central opening. The color of the eye is actually the color of the iris.

1. *Iritis:* Inflammation of the iris and ciliary body (to which the iris is anchored) causes pain, extreme light sensitivity, redness, and a constricted or irregularly shaped pupil.

2. *Heterochromia:* The iris of one eye is different in color than the iris of the other eye. It is usually congenital and harmless. A recent color change is associated with iritis.

3. *Synechiae:* The iris adheres to the lens of the eye producing pain and an irregularly shaped pupil. It usually follows iritis. The iris may sometimes adhere to the back of the cornea following an injury or eye surgery.

4. *Coloboma:* A congenital defect wherein part of the iris is missing. It can also occur after an injury or eye surgery.

5. Tumors and Cysts: Can develop in the iris, ranging from harmless to highly malignant.

6. Iridodonesis: Tremulous iris due to a displaced or missing lens.

II. LENS

Transparent, semi-elastic structure which can change shape to focus at different seeing distances.

1. Subluxated lens: The lens is shifted out of its normal position, usually down. It may be congenital or resulting from an injury. Vision is affected depending on the degree of displacement.

2. Cataract: The lens of the eye becomes cloudy. It is not a growth or film, but a gradual transformation of transparent lens fibers becoming opaque. The most common type is the "senile," associated with aging. The density and location of the opacities will determine the sight loss.

III. VITREOUS

The clear, jelly-like material which fills the inside of the eye behind the lens.

1. Muscae volintantes or Floaters: Small, solidified particles floating in the vitreous which are seen as spots, threads, or specks when looking at a bright background. Harmless, but annoying when in the line of sight.

IV. RETINA

The thin nerve layer covering the inside back of the eye where light is absorbed and converted into electrical signals for sight. Since the retina is profusely supplied with surface blood vessels, general vascular changes can be seen in the eyes.

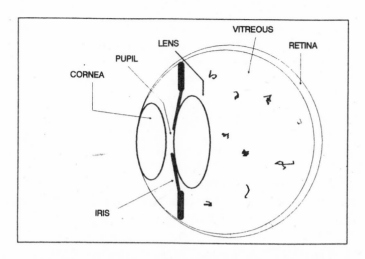

FLOATERS. *Small bits of matter trapped in the vitreous, the clear, jelly-like substance filling the eye behind the lens. They are mostly seen as spots, threads, flies, etc. when looking at a bright background. Generally, it's only an annoying problem which increases with aging as the vitreous becomes somewhat liquefied. Sudden and massive amounts of floaters should be promptly investigated for cause.*

1. *Arteriosclerosis:* The arterial walls become thickened, restricting the blood flow. As the condition worsens, small hemorrhages may occur. A possible serious consequence is an obstruction of a main artery or vein.

2. *Hypertensive retinopathy:* General high blood pressure will, of course, involve the retinal vessels. Besides arteriosclerosis, there may be edema, exudates, and hemorrhages. The sight and extent of retinal damage will determine the sight loss.

3. *Diabetic retinopathy:* Long-standing diabetes will cause engorgement of the veins and the formation of aneurysms. The resulting hemorrhages and exudates will interfere with vision. It is a leading cause of visual impairment.

4. *Arterial/Venous occlusion:*

(a) An obstruction of the central retinal artery or a principal branch, will cause loss of vision either totally (main artery), or in the area supplied by the branch.

(b) An obstruction in a major vein causes massive hemorrhages and sight impairment. As the hemorrhage is slowly absorbed, there is a gradual sight improvement.

5. *Papillitis:* Inflammation of the optic nerve disc.

6. *Papilledema:* The optic nerve disc becomes swollen. The usual cause is an increase in the intracranial pressure and interference with venous circulation of the eye.

7. *Retinitis Pigmentosa:* Degeneration of the retina and gradual loss of side vision. An early symptom of this hereditary disease is night blindness.

8. *Retinal degeneration:* Disturbances in the vascular system will usually lead to degenerative changes. It affects mostly older people with vision gradually being reduced.

9. *Macular degeneration:* Disturbances in the central retinal area (macula), result in sight loss.

10. *Choroiditis:* Inflammation of the choroid which affects the overlying retina. It is caused by a systemic disease which is often difficult to identify. The inflammatory lesions can be at the extreme side with little visual disturbance, or near the macula, with decided sight loss. The inflammation slowly subsides, but repeated attacks are common.

11. *Tumors:* May be malignant or benign. An early symptom may be sight loss due to a retinal detachment.

12. *Retinal detachment:* Any break or tear in the retina can be followed by detachment from the underlying choroid. Possible causes may be a congenital condition, injury, disease, malignant myopia.

V. OPTIC NERVE

The collection of some million individual nerve fibers connecting the eye to the brain.

1. Optic atrophy: The optic nerve fibers are destroyed as a result of disease, injury, or pressure directly on the nerve. Portions of the central and/or side vision are lost.

2. Toxic amblyopia: Loss of central vision due to chronic poisoning, usually tobacco or alcohol.

3. Retrobulbar neuritis: Inflammation of the optic nerve which is usually accompanied by painful eye movements and loss of central vision.

4. Tumors: Any tumors along the nerve pathway will cause a gradual loss of vision, often accompanied by exophthalmos.

VI. ORBIT

The eye is enclosed in a bony vault surrounded with fatty tissue.

1. Inflammation: Bacterial infection of the tissue and fat around the eye.

2. Tumors: A variety of tumors can occur. The most obvious symptoms are a bulging eye and double vision.

3. Exophthalmos: Bulging eyes. When both eyes are involved, the condition is caused by an overactive thyroid. Only one eye bulging is caused by a tumor, inflammation, or vascular condition.

4. Enophthalmos: The appearance of a sunken eyeball. It usually follows an injury or occurs in older people when some of the fatty tissue is absorbed.

VII. GLAUCOMA

Increase in the fluid pressure within the eye causes interference with the blood supply and damage to the sensitive retinal nerves. There is a progressive loss of sight beginning peripherally.

1. Chronic: About 90% of glaucoma is in this category. It has a slow course (many years) without pain and few symptoms in the early stages. Colored halos around lights may be seen on occasion.

2. Acute: This accounts for about 5% of glaucoma. There is a sudden attack of blurred sight, pain, nausea, red eye, and an enlarged immobilized pupil.

3. Secondary: The result of an acquired or congenital eye condition such as an injury, inflammation, degeneration, and some medications (corticosteroids). The resultant glaucoma can be chronic or acute.

43

Allergies and The Eye

An allergy or hypersensitivity can be described as an overreaction by the body's defense/immune system to a specific substance which is normally harmless. (Most people won't react to it.) Although hay fever probably caused sneezing to echo through the forests and caves of our ancestors, there is no doubt that industrialization with its proliferation of artificial products has greatly increased the incidence of allergies. While reactions can occur in any part of the body we will, of course, confine ourselves to the eye and lids.

If you are to suffer an allergic reaction, your system must have been exposed to that substance previously. The first time, there may have been hardly any reaction at all, but a later exposure can cause the immune system to mount an all-out attack against what it perceives to be a threat.

A little background information on the body's immune system will ease your understanding of it's very intricate, multifaceted design. Great strides have been made in the last decade to unravel the mechanism of action, but a great deal is yet to be learned. For our purposes, though, and very briefly, when the immune system encounters anything that it does not recognize as "self", it will produce antibodies against that substance as an initial step to destroy or immobilize it. Any such alien substance that triggers the production of antibodies is called an antigen. When that antigen is linked with a genuinely harmful agent such as bacteria, virus or parasite, you require the immune system to get to work very rapidly and at full power to protect you from harm. However, the immune system, for as yet unknown reasons, can sometimes attack normal body cells. If this happens it causes autoimmune diseases such as rheumatoid arthritis or multiple sclerosis. The immune system can also organize a large attack which is way out of proportion to a mild threat—the allergic reaction.

When does an antigen also become an allergen to provoke an allergic reaction? When it has the correct molecular size to interact with mast cells. These mast cells are one of the immune system's arsenal of weapons. They are exceptionally numerous in the conjunctiva of the eye (about 50 million per eye), and are the prime instigators in the process. Allergens act on the mast cells to swiftly release histamines for the immediate allergic reaction. But the process doesn't stop there. The mast cells also release other substances which then synthesize proteins for longer lasting inflammatory responses and tissue damage. Ultimately, the tissue is primed for the next antigen like a dynamite fuse waiting to be lighted.

Common Allergens

Airborne particles that you inhale are the most common route to allergic reactions and typically affect the eyes with itching, redness, tearing and swelling. They include plant pollen, fungal spores, animal danders, and house dust. Actually, it's not the dust itself, but very tiny mites which live in pillows, mattresses, carpets, etc. It's probably not possible to get rid of them and you may suffer year-round. Pollen allergies, on the other hand, will be seasonal.

Some people are allergic to certain foods (eggs, fish, nuts, milk), but these rarely concern the eyes. A variety of drugs can cause allergic reactions, penicillin being a well-known example, and some will cause eye symptoms.

The eyes are very prone to allergic reactions from direct contact with specific substances. Pet your pet and touch your lids and you may get red, itchy eyes. The use of makeup is a familiar problem. Some contact lens wearers develop allergies to the solutions used for cleaning or storage.

Allergic Conjunctivitis

Conjunctivitis is an inflammation of the conjunctiva, the thin, transparent covering on the white of the eye and the inside of the lids. It can be caused by bacteria or a virus, but we'll only discuss the main allergic types.

Hay Fever, Rose Fever: If you don't have it, you know someone who does—it's so widespread. The pollen from trees, grasses, etc. cause tearing, itching, light sensitivity and burning. There is generally a very strong family history of these allergies. The primary treatment is to remove the allergenic substances, which is much easier said than done. Useful treatment medications include topical vasoconstrictors which decreases the amount of histamines, etc. by constricting the small blood vessels. Oral antihistamines, and occasionally mild steroids may also be necessary. The chronic use of a vasoconstrictor could cause an increase of symptoms if you become allergic to the ingredients.

Contact Conjunctivitis: This will usually develop a day or several days after exposure to cosmetics, poison ivy, soaps, eye medication, etc. The skin of the lids is puffy and red; the eyes are itchy and burning. The first step is to eliminate the triggering substance, although it may take time to figure out which product is the culprit. If you suspect eye makeup, stop using everything for a few days until all symptoms are gone. Then gradually begin using one product at a time at intervals of 4 to 5 days, and you may be able to pinpoint the offending ingredient. For treating the symptoms, try cold compresses 2 to 4 times a day. Your doctor may also prescribe medication.

Giant Papillary Conjunctivitis (GPC): This is a relatively "new" disease in the sense that it is caused by wearing contact lenses, especially soft lenses and more especially, extended wear lenses. The gradual buildup of protein material (natural eye secretions) on the lens surfaces creates an immunologic response on the inner surface of the upper lid in susceptible people. Albeit it's your own protein on the lenses, it is not considered an autoimmune process because the protein becomes denatured, i.e., changes its structure. Small papilla (bumps) develop on the inside of the upper lid. In the early stages, discontinuing contact lens wear, replacing the lenses with lenses made of a different polymer material, reducing the wearing time, and conscientiously cleaning the lenses should all keep the condition under control. Topical eye drops can be prescribed to offer relief.

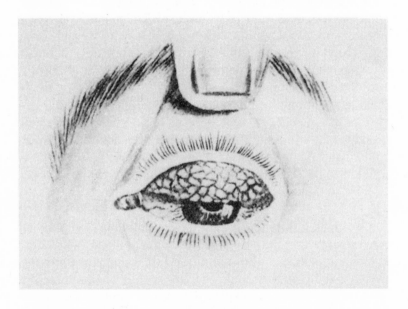

Inverting the upper lid to show giant papillary conjunctivitis.

Once it has reached an advanced stage with larger, more numerous bumps there is itching, discharge, discomfort, and the contact lens will be displaced by the thickened lid. Contact lens wear has to be discontinued to remove the source of the allergen. Topical antihistamines and/or vasoconstrictors are helpful along with artificial tear ointments. Resuming contact lens wear is questionable. An important point to understand is that simply not wearing contact lenses will gradually decrease the symptoms (because the allergen source is eliminated.) GPC does not seem to cause any damage to the cornea or vision.

Vernal Conjunctivitis: The word vernal means spring and this ailment usually occurs and recurs in the warmer months of temperate climates. Recurs is an apt adjective because it usually strikes young children, abates during cold weather, returns in warm weather, lasts from 4 to 10 years, and hardly ever affects someone over 25 years of age. Boys are twice as vulnerable as girls. The symptoms include considerable itching, burning, stringy discharge, light sensitivity. The inside of the upper lid develops bumps not unlike GPC. The cornea may also be involved.

Remaining in cool surroundings as much as possible seems to help. Steroids afford some relief but the long course of the disease makes it unacceptable to continue steroids indefinitely for fear of the side effects. A way around this is to go on and off steroids at intervals.

Corneal Allergic Reactions: The cornea may become involved in allergic reactions which are usually more serious than conjunctival reactions. A typical reaction can be from medications instilled in the eye. The cornea may also react to toxins produced by certain bacteria such as Treponema pallidus (causes syphilis) and staphylococcus. Often a corneal specialist needs to be consulted.

44

Drugs Affecting Eyes and Vision

Modern medicine relies heavily on the hundreds of drugs available to the physician to control or banish diseases. We can hardly imagine life without pills, injections, serums, tonics, etc. However, you must remember the basic principal that ALL medication has some side effect. The second principal is that not all side effects touch everyone. The challenge for the physician is to balance the potential benefit against the possible harm it can induce.

The Food and Drug Administration is mandated to investigate all new drugs for effectiveness and adverse reactions. The very occasional and very unfortunate slip-ups make the headlines, and sometimes the length and complexity of the approval process is disparaged. There is always conflicting pressure from those people who want the product brought quickly to market and those who want more testing for safety. Overall, considering that the FDA is a government bureaucracy (which can always benefit from improvements), that agency does reasonably well in a difficult capacity.

It's a simple fact of life that with aging comes a greater dependence on medication for such things a elevated blood pressure, heart conditions, arthritis, etc. With most of these conditions, the drug treatment will be ongoing and open-ended which increases the risk of unwanted side effects. But even limited use of certain powerful drugs can have adverse affects. Approximately 3–4% of these reactions affect the vision or cause damage to parts of the eye. They may begin shortly after starting a drug or after prolonged use. Some reactions are minor, subtle affects such as blurring, lid swelling, difficulty reading. More pronounced symptoms include double vision, light sensitivity or nystagmus. In severe reactions retinal hemorrhages, optic nerve damage or glaucoma may result.

The following guide notes the possible reactions for the eyes and vision only; there will likely also be reactions affecting other parts of the body. We have listed the most common and widely employed pharmaceuticals and the uses for which they are generally prescribed. You must be aware that if you are taking more than one medication they can interact to yield serious side affects. For complete information on the medicine you're using, ask your physician.

GENERIC ACTIVE INGREDIENT	BRAND NAME	USED FOR	OCULAR SIDE EFFECTS
Acetaminophen	Tylenol/Codeine	Analgesic for mild to moderate pain	Pinpoint pupil. Visual disturbances.
Acetazolamide	Diamox	Immunization under age 7	Nearsightedness. Blurred vision.
Allopurinol	Zyloprim	Gout	Cataracts? Visual disturbances.
Alcohol	Alcohol		Difficulty controlling eye movements.
Alpha-Methyl-Dopa	Aldomet	Hypertension	Rare.
Amiloride HCL	Moduretic	Hypertension and edema	Visual disturbances. Color vision changes.
Amiodarone	Cordarone	Smooth heart rhythm	Corneal changes. Cataracts.
Amitriptyline	Elavil	Antidepressant	Double vision. Reading difficulty.
Amoxicillion	Amoxil	Infections	Few.
Atenolol	Tenormin	Hypertension	Dry eyes. Visual disturbances.
Butalbital	Fiorinal	Tension headaches	Rare.
Chlordiazepoxide	Librium	Anxiety; tension	Rare.
Chloroquine	Atabrine HCL	Malaria	Corneal changes. Visual field loss. Color vision changes. Double vision.
Chlorpheniramine	Chlor-Trimeton	Allergies	Dry eyes. Enlarged pupils.
Chlorpromazine	Thorazine	Psychotic disorders	Discoloration of sclera. Double vision. Cataracts. Vision impairment. Cornea.
Chlorpropamide	Diabinese	Mild diabetes	Few.
Cimetidine	Tagamet	Duodenal ulcer	Rare.
Clonidine	Catapres	Hypertension	Rare.
Clorazepate dipotassium	Tranxene	Antianxiety Alcohol withdrawal	Decreased focusing, depth perception.
Codeine	See Tylenol/Codeine		
Corticosteroid	Prednisone	Inflammation	Cataracts. Raises eye pressure.
Diazepam	Valium	Antianxiety Alcohol withdrawal	Rare.
Digoxin	Lanoxin	Congestive heart failure	Frequent color vision changes. Halos. Double vision. Glare.
Diphenhydramine HCL	Benadryl	Allergies Motion sickness	Visual disburbances. Double vision. Enlarged pupils.

GENERIC ACTIVE INGREDIENT	BRAND NAME	USED FOR	OCULAR SIDE EFFECTS
Dipyridamole	Persantine	Angina	Few.
Erythromycin	E.E.S.	Infections	Few. Color vision.
Estrogen	Premarin	Menopause	Corneal curvature, visual changes. Intolerance to contact lenses.
Ethambutol	Myambutol	Tuberculosis	Optic nerve changes. Light sensitivity.
Ethinyl estradiol	Ortho-Novum	Oral contraceptive	Optic neuritis. Retinal thrombosis. Loss of vision. Double vision.
Flurazapam HCL	Dalmane	Insomnia	Decreased vision, focusing, depth perception. Dilated pupil. Glaucoma.
Flurosemide	Lasix	Hypertension	Rare.
Hydrochlorothiazide	Dyazide	Hypertension; angina; migraine	Rare.
Hyoscyamine	Donnatal	Peptic ulcer	Blurred vision. Light sensitivity. Glaucoma. Enlarged pupils. Reading difficulty.
Ibuprofen	Motrin	Arthritis	Visual disturbances. Double vision.
Indomethacin	Indocin	Arthritis	Visual disturbances. Double vision.
Isosorbide dinitrate	Isordil	Angina	Rare.
Isotretinoin	Accutane	Severe acne	Retinal changes. Dry eyes. Light sensitivity. Conjunctivitis.
Levothyroxine sodium	Synthroid	Thyroid replacement	Rare.
Lithium		Psychic disorders	Blurred vision. Double vision. Dry eyes. Contact lens intolerance.
Lorazapam	Ativan	Antianxiety; insomnia	Blurred vision. Double vision.
Lovastatin	Mevacor	High cholesterol	Blurred vision.
Meclizine HCL	Antivert	Motion sickness	Rare.
Methoxsalen	Oxsoralen	Psoriasis; vitiligo	Cataracts.
Metranol	Ortho-Novum	Oral contraceptive	Optic neuritis. Retinal thrombosis. Double vision.
Metroprolol tartrate	Lopressor	Hypertension	Dry eyes. Blurred vision.
Nadolol	Corgard	Hypertension; angina	Rare.
Naproxen	Naprosyn	Arthritis	Blurred vision. Double vision. Optic neuritis.
Nifedipine	Procardia	Angina	Few.

GENERIC ACTIVE INGREDIENT	BRAND NAME	USED FOR	OCULAR SIDE EFFECTS
Nitroglycerin	Nitrostat	Angina	Rare.
Norethindrone	Ortho-Novum	Oral contraceptive	Optic neuritis. Retinal thrombosis. Double vision.
Norgestrel	Lo/Ovral	Oral contraceptive	Corneal curvature changes. Contact lens intolerance.
Phenobarbital	Donnatal	Peptic ulcer	Blurred vision. Light sensitivity. Increased intraocular pressure. Dilated pupils.
Phenylephrine HCL Phenylpropanolomine HCL	Triaminic; Dimetapp	Cold remedy	Dry eyes. Reduced contact lens wear.
Phenytoin	Dilantin	Grand mal; seizures	Nystagmus. Double vision. Reading difficulty.
Piroxicam	Feldene	Arthritis	Rare.
Prozasin HCL	Minipress	Hypertension	Blurred vision. Red eyes.
Propanolol HCL	Inderal	Hypertension; angina	Rare.
Scopolamine	Donnatal	Peptic ulcer	Blurred vision. Light sensitivity. Dilated pupils. Reading difficulty.
Spironolactone	Aldactazide	Hypertension	Visual disturbances. Color vision changes. Nearsightedness.
Sulindac	Clinoril	Arthritis	Blurred vision. Retinal degeneration. Conjunctivitis.
Tamoxifen	Nolvadex	Breast cancer	Retinal changes. Corneal changes. Cataracts.
Temazepam	Restoril	Insomnia	Rare.
Terbutalinc sulfaic	Brethine	Bronchial asthma	Rare.
Theophyline	Theo-Dur, Slo-Bid	Asthma	Rare.
Tolazamide	Tolinase	Diabetes	Rare.
Triamterene	Dyazide; Maxzide	Hypertension; edema	Rare.
Warfarin sodium	Coumadin	Thrombosis; emboli	Dry eyes. Visual disturbances. Color vision changes.

45

Symptoms and Complaints

When you report a symptom or physical complaint to your doctor, it brings certain possible causes to his or her mind. They can range from minor irregularities requiring no treatment, to serious ailments requiring prompt attention. This chapter will acquaint you with the causes of many of your symptoms and complaints. With the help of the section on Common Eye Diseases and Disorders, you may be able to tentatively diagnose some, but most require professional judgment. As a word of caution—don't make the error of the beginning medical student and consider every slight symptom a sign of a fatal affliction.

Where it applies, we have clearly indicated both the common and infrequent causes of symptoms and complaints in each category.

Blurred Vision

   I. When looking at distance
      Common:
         (a) Nearsighted

    (b) Astigmatism

    (c) Farsighted (depending on amount and age)

Infrequent:

    (a) Cataracts

    (b) Diabetes

    (c) Amblyopia

    (d) Drug reactions

    (e) Diseases of eye or brain

    (f) Congenital, hereditary abnormalities

    (g) Spasm of focusing muscles

II. When looking at near

Common:

    (a) Farsighted

    (b) Astigmatism

    (c) Presbyopia (gradual failure of focusing ability with aging)

Infrequent:

    (a) Cataracts

    (b) Diabetes

    (c) Drug reactions

    (d) Congenital, hereditary abnormalities

    (e) Diseases of the eye or brain

    (f) Fatigue of convergence skill

Night Blindness

The usual complaint of poor vision at night is not actually night blindness. It is a difficulty in seeing or walking around in dim light. This could be caused by:

    (a) Loss of contrast sensitivity with aging or from circulatory problems

    (b) A person's exact "dark focus"

    (c) Overexposure to bright sunlight during the day

    (d) Drugs (especially alcohol and tobacco)

True night blindness is a rare disease; there is a total inability to see in dim light.

Common:

    (a) Vitamin A deficiency

    (b) Retinal degeneration

Infrequent:
- (a) Advanced glaucoma
- (b) Diseases of optic nerve
- (c) Psychic disorders

Distorted Vision

Objects appear to be misshaped or different in size.

Common:
- (a) Swelling or inflammation at back of eye

Infrequent:
- (a) Drug reactions (including excessive use of alcohol, tobacco)
- (b) During migraine headache attack
- (c) Retinal detachment
- (d) Neurological or brain disorders
- (e) Psychic disorders

Temporary Blindness

Generally only one eye is involved. It can last from a few seconds, to hours or even days.

Common:
- (a) Blockage of blood supply to eye or brain
- (b) Psychic disorder (hysteria)

Infrequent:
- (a) Poisoning
- (b) Injury
- (c) Drug reaction (including excessive use of alcohol, tobacco)
- (d) Neurological or brain disorders.

Central Vision Loss

Direct, straight ahead sight is poor, while peripheral (side) vision is retained.

Common:
- (a) Macular Degeneration
- (b) Reduced blood supply or hemorrhage
- (c) Swelling or edema of macula

Infrequent:
- (a) Amblyopia
- (b) Drug reactions
- (c) Hereditary
- (d) Retinal damage as a result of excessive infrared radiation (from welding, looking at an eclipse, etc.)
- (e) Inflammation
- (f) Neurological disorders
- (g) Cysts, tumors
- (h) Retinal detachment

Side Vision Loss

Either one or both eyes can be involved. The loss may only be in a small area, the right or left half of the visual field, or the entire field.

Sudden onset:
- (a) Retinal detachment
- (b) Reduced blood supply or hemorrhage
- (c) Swelling or edema

Gradual loss:
- (a) Retinal degeneration
- (b) Glaucoma
- (c) Hereditary
- (d) Injury
- (e) Neurological, brain diseases and disorders
- (f) Inflammation or disease of optic nerve

Light Flashes

Common:
- (a) Hardening of the arteries or other blood supply disturbances

Infrequent:
- (a) Severe coughing or sneezing
- (b) May precede retinal detachment
- (c) May precede migraine or epilepsy attack
- (d) Drug reactions
- (e) Brain concussion
- (f) Irritation to retina or optic nerve
- (g) Rubbing or pressing on eyes
- (h) Inflammation or infection of retina

Double Vision

Seeing two objects when there is really only one. The two objects may be seen next to each other, above each other, or at an angle.

I. When seen with one eye
  Common:
    (a) Lens or corneal abnormalities
  Infrequent:
    (a) Astigmatism
    (b) Torn iris
    (c) Disease or injury to cornea
    (d) Displaced lens
    (e) Early cataract changes
    (f) Psychic disorders

II. When seen with two eyes
  Common:
    (a) Paralysis of one or more of the muscles controlling eye movements
    (b) Imbalance in action of muscles controlling eye movements
  Infrequent:
    (a) Drug reactions
    (b) Aniseikonia
    (c) Neurological and brain disorders
    (d) Following eye or brain surgery

Floating Spots

Seen as spots, threads, or specks against a bright background.
  Common:
    (a) Solidified particles in vitreous, usually in older people. Quite harmless.
  Infrequent:
    (a) Inflammation
    (b) Hemorrhage in retina
    (c) May precede retinal detachment

Light Sensitivity

I. Severe

Common:

(a) Foreign particle on eye

(b) Injury to cornea

Infrequent:

(a) Inflammation

(b) Drug reaction

(c) Hereditary (such as albinism)

(d) Enlarged pupil which doesn't constrict to light

II. Mild

Common:

(a) Inflammation of lids or eye

(b) Contact lens wear

Infrequent:

(a) Neuralgia, neuritis

(b) Migraine headaches

(c) Focusing effort fatigue

(d) Dental problems

(e) Extreme nearsightedness

(f) Drug reactions or poisoning

Halos Around Lights

Rings of colors or halos around light sources. One or both eyes can be affected.

Common:

(a) Glaucoma

(b) Swelling of cornea (often from contact lens overwear)

(c) Cataracts

Infrequent:

(a) Corneal scar

(b) Disease of cornea

(c) Drug reactions

Pain in Eye

I. Moderate to severe

Common:
- (a) Foreign particle on cornea or lids
- (b) Inflammation in or around the eye

Infrequent:
- (a) Inverted eyelash
- (b) Acute glaucoma (usually with nausea)
- (c) Corneal abrasion from wearing contact lenses too long or from poor fitting contact lenses
- (d) Neuralgia (usually one side of face)
- (e) Disease or injury to cornea
- (f) Sinus infection

II. Discomfort, eye strain, or dull ache

Common:
- (a) Farsighted
- (b) Astigmatism
- (c) Presbyopia
- (d) Imbalance of action of muscles controlling eye movements
- (e) Fatigue of focusing or eye convergence (usually in afternoon after close work)

Infrequent:
- (a) Chronic conjunctivitis
- (b) Light glare; too much or too little light
- (c) Lack of sleep or rest
- (d) Aniseikonia

III. Sensation of burning, itching, smarting

Common:
- (a) Conjunctivitis
- (b) Allergies

Infrequent:
- (a) Drug reactions
- (b) Dry eyes
- (c) Contact lens wear
- (d) Atmosphere conditions and pollutants

Headaches

I. Associated with the use of the eyes

Common:
- (a) Farsighted
- (b) Astigmatism
- (c) Imbalance of action of muscles controlling eye movements
- (d) Fatigue of focusing or eye convergence (usually after prolonged close work)

Infrequent:
- (a) Aniseikonia

II. Not associated with use of the eyes
Common:
- (a) Neuralgia (usually one side of head)
- (b) Sinus infection
- (c) High or low blood pressure
- (d) General fatigue
- (e) Too much alcohol, overeating, etc.
- (f) General disease or infection
- (g) Migraine (one side of head)

Redness

I. Lids
Common:
- (a) Styes
- (b) Allergies
- (c) Conjunctivitis

Infrequent:
- (a) Insect bite
- (b) Blocked tear duct
- (c) Inflammation of any of the numerous lid glands

II. Eye
Common:
- (a) Hemorrhage of small blood vessel from injury or disease (shows up dramatically against white of eye)
- (b) Inflammation or disease
- (c) Acute conjunctivitis

Infrequent:
- (a) Acute glaucoma

Secretions and Discharges

I. Excessive tearing

Common:
- (a) Irritation to cornea
- (b) Allergies
- (c) Wind or cold weather
- (d) Blocked tear drainage system
- (e) In older people, loose lower lid
- (f) Psychological

Infrequent:
- (a) Inflammation
- (b) Bright light or glare
- (c) Chemical irritants
- (d) Poorly fitting contact lenses
- (e) Disease of tear gland
- (f) Imbalance of muscles controlling eye movements
- (g) Reading strain

II. Unusual discharges (pus, mucous, etc.)

Common:
- (a) Conjunctivitis
- (b) Allergies
- (c) Inflammation of lid margin

Infrequent:
- (a) Dry eyes
- (b) Infections
- (c) Inflammation of lid glands
- (d) Chemical irritants

Frequent Blinking

Common:
- (a) Together with a facial tic, a habit in some children

Infrequent:
- (a) Older people with dry eyes
- (b) Nervous system disease

Change In Pupil Size

I. Dilated (large)

Common:
- (a) In dim light
- (b) Drug reactions

    (c) Disease or injury to nervous system

    (d) Psychological (pleasure, fear, etc.)

Infrequent:

    (a) Glaucoma

    (b) Tumors of brain

    (c) Coma as from diabetes, epilepsy, etc.

    (d) Diseases of the retina

II. Constricted (small)

Common:

    (a) In bright light

    (b) Normal condition in older people

    (c) Drug reactions (including too much alcohol)

Infrequent:

    (a) General diseases such as syphilis, diabetes, multiple sclerosis

    (b) Diseases of central nervous system

    (c) Psychological

Small Lumps

I. Lids

Common:

    (a) Sty (Swelling near lid margin growing into small lump. Comes to a yellowish head, breaks open and discharges matter. Heals quickly.

    (b) Cysts

Infrequent:

    (a) Tumors and fatty tissue accumulation

II. Eye

Common:

    (a) Cysts

    (b) Fatty deposits

Infrequent:

    (a) Tumors

Colored Spots On White Of Eye

Common:

    (a) Pigmented tumors

    (b) Small blood vessel loops

    (c) Pinguecula

    (d) Small hemorrhage

Infrequent:
- (a) Inflammation
- (b) Vitamin A deficiency
- (c) Drug reactions
- (d) Thinned areas of white cover tissue
- (e) After eye surgery

Eyelids

I. Droopy. Generally only one lid is affected
Common:
- (a) Hereditary
- (b) With aging, loss of muscle tone and decrease of fatty tissue

Infrequent:
- (a) Paralyzed lid muscle
- (b) Neurological disorder
- (c) General diseases
- (d) Tumors
- (e) Hemorrhage
- (f) Insect bite (temporary swelling may give appearance of droop)
- (g) After lid or eye surgery

II. Swelling
Common:
- (a) Allergies
- (b) Inflammation
- (c) Problems with blood supply

Infrequent:
- (a) Insect bite
- (b) Infections
- (c) Reactions to vaccines, penicillin, etc.
- (d) Swollen tear gland
- (e) Tumors
- (f) Injury

III. Baggy (loose folds of skin)
- (a) Hereditary
- (b) Weight loss

IV. Margins turn inward or outward
- (a) Congenital
- (b) Allergies

    (c) Aging process

    (d) Scar tissue

    (e) Spasm of lid muscles

Protruding Eyeball

  I. When both eyes are involved

    Common:

      (a) Overactive thyroid

  II. When one eye is involved

      (a) Swelling

      (b) Inflammation

      (c) Tumors

      (d) Injury

Shrinking Eyeball

Generally, the eyeball is not getting smaller, but only gives that appearance because the fatty tissue around the globe is diminishing.

    (a) In aged persons

    (b) Following cataract surgery

    (c) Injury

A true sunken eyeball is blind.

    (a) Congenital

    (b) Disease

    (c) Injury

    (d) Tumors

Eye Oscillations

The rapid movements may be back and forth, up and down, or mixed

    Common:

      (a) Congenital

    Infrequent:

      (a) Diseases of the brain and nervous system

      (b) Tumors of the brain and nervous system

46

Common Ophthalmic Medical Conditions & Treatments

I t may surprise you to learn there are about two hundred conditions which can afflict the eyes, lids, surrounding tissues and structures. Of that large number, about a dozen could be labeled common and most often encountered in an optometrist's office. Those are the ones we will cover here. As you read this chapter, it will become apparent that many of these conditions have similar and overlapping symptoms. While it might be intellectually interesting and challenging to attempt a self diagnosis, you will probably be wrong. If you are, and delay treatment, it could lead to sight threatening complications.

The Red Eye

The ubiquitous "pink eye" or "red eye" is the most well-known external eye condition simply because it's so very conspicuous. It stands out more than the proverbial sore thumb. Almost everyone has either had it at one time or another or has been in close contact with someone who did. But what is it?

Describing the eye as "pink" or "red" really says nothing about the condition except that the eye is not its normal white. Many things can cause the eye or lids to redden. Some are merely an annoyance; others could be sight threatening. Some are self-limiting within a few days; others are highly contagious and spread to family members. Some require mild supportive therapy; others require vigorous medical intervention. The stock feature is that the blood vessels within the normally white of the eye become engorged in response to distress signals from the tissue under siege. This is not just a casual or offhand response. It's a very vital and practical action to bring the immune system's arsenal of weapons to the site. In other words, the redness means an inflammation is going on which is the way the body normally copes with anything it perceives as a threat to itself. The dilated blood vessels not only bring a greater volume of blood to the location, but also become more permeable (leaky) so that the army of cells and infection-fighting substances in the blood can filter into the tissue and be brought to bear on the "invasion."

For the external eye, in medical terms, this is generally a conjunctivitis — an inflammation of the conjunctiva which is the thin, transparent membrane lining the "white" of the eye and the inside of the lids. The same inflammation process takes place in other parts of the body but is far less obvious than underneath the translucent tissue of the eye. (If your finger gets inflamed, the redness is moderated by the nearly opaque skin and you become aware of it principally by the pain/tenderness.) Let's sort out the various types of possible conjunctivitis conditions and discuss treatment options.

What can produce an inflammation? An allergic reaction, infection, injury or very dry eyes, which is really an injury in progress. The majority of conjunctivitis cases are allergic or viral. (However, the number of dry eye patients being seen is becoming quite large and dry eyes are often associated with the other conditions.) Reading Chapter 43, Allergies and the Eye, will give you the framework, but because allergic conditions are so commonplace, we'll go into more detail in the treatment options currently available.

Allergic

The principal symptoms of allergic conjunctivitis are redness, itching, swelling and some watery or mucus discharge. For most people, itching is the most miserable thing to deal with. The simplest way to dodge an allergic reaction, of course, is to avoid the substance causing it. You might be able to change your eye makeup to a non-allergic type or refrain from petting a cat, but can you really avoid pollen or dust?

The majority of people with allergic conjunctivitis (about eight out of ten) suffer from hay fever or other seasonal allergies. If the symptoms are mild, they can be managed with topical eye drops of a decongestant/astringent combination such as Vasoclear or Zincfrin, two to four times a day. These are available without a prescription. If the itching is fairly severe, a vasoconstrictor/antihistamine combination drop is more effective. Some brand names currently available over-the-counter: Naphcon-A, Vasocon-A and Albalon-A. These may have to be augmented by an oral antihistamine such as Chlor-Trimeton or Benadryl, two or three times a day.

If you fit into the roughly half of the allergic population which does not get relief from these modest measures, you may require a more powerful prescription medication. In the last few years, a number of effective drugs have become available to subdue many previously stubborn allergic symptoms. In extremely unresponsive cases, steroid eye drops must also be prescribed

This might be a good place to specify the proper way to use any topical eye medication. You need to be sure the medication is stored properly, is not past the expiration date, and has not become contaminated.

Installation of Eye Drops

• Wash your hands before and after using eye medication.
• Tilt your head back and look up at the ceiling or you can lie down on your back if it's easier.

• Place a finger on your cheek just <u>under</u> your lower eyelid and gently pull down until a **V** pocket is formed between your eyeball and your lower lid.

• Put the drop into the eye. To avoid contaminating the dropper, do not let the tip touch your eye or lashes. The eyeball can only hold one drop. Putting in more is a waste.

• Do <u>not</u> blink. Simply close your eyes gently and leave them closed for a minute.

Installation of Ointment

• Same as above except place a small amount, about 1/4-inch ribbon, of ointment into the **V** pocket.

• Do <u>not</u> let the tip of the tube touch your eye or eyelashes.

INFECTIVE CONJUNCTIVITIS

As the name implies, some microbe has set up an infection in the eye. Where do the microbes come from? Just like your skin, the inside of your mouth, nose, etc., the eyes and lids are literally coated with a variety of bacteria, virus, molds and other denizens of the microscopic world. The intact skin is a good protective barrier. If you cut your finger and disrupt that barrier, an infection process can begin. As far as the eyes and lids are concerned, most of the microbe population is harmless and the immune system via the tears and other defensive tactics can generally deal effectively to keep them under a safe level of control. Sometimes, however, there is an eruption of microbe numbers, multiplying too rapidly for the immune system to overcome. Or you may touch a source of infection and then touch or rub your eye transferring the "bad" guys to yourself. They set up shop, multiply, and an infection and inflammation soon follow.

Think of it in terms of a school lunchroom where there is always a low level of tumult and disorder which the staff can easily handle and keep under control. But sometimes a serious fight might erupt and then additional help has to be brought in (maybe the football coach) to quell the disturbance. If school gangs are involved ("bad" microbes) the situation can take on a dangerous aspect and may even become chronic with periods of relative calm punctuated by periods of disturbances.

Infective conjunctivitis can be caused by a virus, bacteria, a fungus or a parasite. The last two are extremely difficult to deal with and fortunately do not fall into the "common" condition category except in some underdeveloped countries where they are a serious health problem.

<u>Viral conjunctivitis</u> may follow an upper respiratory infection or contact with someone who already has it. There are many different viruses which can infect the eye and cause the symptoms of redness, burning, irritation and watering. Just as there is no treatment for the common viral cold, there is no anti-viral medication for viral conjunctivitis. In mild conditions, treatment revolves around calming the symptoms as much as possible with artificial tears, cool compresses and a vasoconstrictor/antihistamine if itching is a problem. This is a very contagious disease and will easily spread via hand touching, using the same towel, etc. From time to time, epidemic outbreaks will occur in children and young adults because of the highly contagious nature. In severe cases, steroid drops and/or non steroidal anti-inflammatory medications may be necessary.

How to Use Cool Compresses

• Use a glycol pack. That's the type you put into the freezer to chill.

• Apply the pack to the closed eyes for one or two minutes with a 10-second break for a total of five minutes.

• Do this four to five times a day for one week.

Like the common cold, the symptoms worsen for about a week, then gradually ease off in the next two to three weeks. Unfortunately, the cornea sometimes becomes involved in the inflammatory process. Certain immune system cells will infiltrate into the clear cornea forming clumps of tiny grayish spots. If these accumulate in the center of the cornea, vision can be affected. A topical steroid is prescribed to dissipate the spots, but it can be a lengthy treatment which takes many months.

The common <u>bacterial conjunctivitis</u> can produce mild redness, swelling, tearing, discharge, and small bumps on the inside of the lids. The doctor will try to differentiate between the various causative organisms, which is sometimes a problem. Smears and cultures can be obtained to make a definite diagnosis, and in a perfect world this would be done. However, the time and expense are generally not indicated unless the bacterial infection doesn't respond to normal antibiotic treatment. "Normal" means that a broad-spectrum antibiotic is prescribed which should deal with the majority of probable bacteria. If the infection doesn't retreat in a few days, then a culture may be needed or the doctor may switch you to an antibiotic with different properties.

True "pink" eye is a <u>severe bacterial conjunctivitis</u> which develops very rapidly with all the above symptoms but more intense. This type is very contagious and will quickly spread to the other eye as well as other family members via contact, towels or hands. Topical antimicrobial drugs are indicated. Great care needs to be taken to avoid spreading the infection to others in the family.

SUBCONJUNCTIVAL HEMORRHAGE

This is one of those conditions which most of the time looks much worse than it really is (like the dog whose bark is worse than the bite). You look in the mirror and are shocked to see a large bloody area where the eye is supposed to be white. What has happened is that one of the small, usually unnoticed blood vessels within the sclera has ruptured painlessly and the escaped blood "pools" under the clear tissue of the eye. This is sometimes associated with high blood pressure, but often it can be triggered by vigorous rubbing of the eye, a coughing fit or just a "spontaneous" action. As awful as it looks, no treatment is needed or satisfactory. The blood will gradually be absorbed over a span of about a week.

LID INFECTIONS

The familiar stye - external hordeolum - is an acute bacterial (staphylococcus) infection of an eyelash follicle or sweat and oil glands along the lid margin. At first you'll feel some tenderness of the lid when blinking and certainly when you touch it. The tenderness and eventual pain are caused by the swelling of the tissue in the inflammation process. Over a period of a couple of days, the area will come to a "head," break open and the pus will drain. To speed the process along, warm, moist compresses should be applied several times a day. In addition, an antibiotic ointment is advisable to prevent further infection. If the offending lash follicle can be located by the doctor, it should be removed to allow quicker drainage.

A stye on the *inside* of the lid is less common but also less likely to readily resolve by itself. Treatment, the same as for a stye on the outside, is usually necessary.

A CHALAZION begins life looking like a stye on the inside of the lid, but doesn't come to a "head." Instead, it may grow very slowly to a round nodule. Moist, warm compresses four times a day with an antibiotic ointment may gradually cause it to diminish and disappear. Unless it becomes very large, it rarely causes vision problems, only a cosmetic concern. If the chalazion is a cosmetic embarrassment, a drug injection can shrink it or it can be removed surgically.

BLEPHARITIS is a stubborn, generally chronic inflammation of the eyelid margins. The lids are red, itchy, with pain and a burning sensation. There are three types: seborrheic, staphylococcal, and mixed.

Seborrheic goes along with a scaly skin condition of the scalp and eyebrows. The scales attached to the eyelashes can be removed with hot compresses. An ongoing program of lid hygiene is needed to keep it under control. This consists of daily scrubbing the lid margins with a gauze pad or a cotton-tip applicator dipped in a special eyelid cleanser or baby shampoo. Because this is a chronic condition, the lid scrubbing must be done faithfully. Many people get tired of the routine after a while and the blepharitis will flare up again.

A more serious blepharitis is caused by a bacterial infection. This is a very frustrating disease to deal with because it's difficult to achieve a cure. Depending on the severity, there is redness, pain, light sensitivity, tearing and blurred vision. Scales of skin form around the lashes. When they are lifted off, there could be ulceration at the base of the lashes. Styes and chalazia occur frequently. The lashes may be damaged or missing altogether. Sometimes the cornea is involved from the toxins produced by the bacteria.

The disease has a tendency to cycle with flare ups between relatively quiet times. Lid hygiene is important but is not sufficient to tame this condition and antibiotic ointments are needed for months. Sometimes, oral antibiotics must also be taken to quiet a flare up.

DRY EYES

While this condition sounds rather benign, the complaints of eyes which feel "gritty," "burning," "hurting," "tired" and/or "watery" and "teary" are heard more often than any others from patients in the optometrist's office. The symptoms may wax and wane depending on the season of the year and the amount of moisture in the air. The cause could be inadequate tear production by glands in the lids and/or rapid evaporation. An additional aggravating factor could be medications being taken for a variety of conditions. These would include a diverse group such as antihistamines, anti-anxiety drugs, diuretics and beta-blockers for high blood pressure, and oral contraceptives. Arthritis, acne rosacea and sarcoidosis are some of the systemic diseases which can also cause dry eyes. For women, menopause often magnifies dryness. Older people are more prone to dry eyes simply because aging reduces the amount of tears produced and can adversely alter the ingredients of the normal film of tears on the eyes. (Chapter 12 has a section explaining the tear film.)

So what if the tear film is diminished? You have to understand that the tears have three vital functions: 1) The cornea must be kept moist or it will lose its transparency; 2) foreign particles and allergy causing substances are rinsed away; 3) components in the tears will disable many microbes. From the last two it should be obvious that dry eyes are a contributing factor for allergic reactions and infections.

You may have caught the apparent contradictory complaint mentioned above - watery and teary eyes. How can the eye be dry if it waters? The explanation is simple. A dry eye will trigger reflex tearing such as when crying. These tears are too dilute to keep the eye moist for very long and don't accomplish the job of lubricating the eye.

Like many conditions, dry eyes can be anything from a mild annoyance to considerable discomfort. There is no known "cure." Relief can only be obtained with an ongoing fare of moisturizing the eyes. Many artificial tear products are available in many degrees of viscosity. Your doctor will recommend a particular class and/or brand. Regardless of the specific eye drops, there are a number of things to keep in mind. It's important, especially when you first start the therapy, to use the drops frequently — every couple of hours. You can't really use them too often, but it's advisable to obtain preservative-free drops to avoid an allergic reaction to a preservative chemical. These preservative-free drops come in tiny plastic vials which can be used for one day. One drug company has developed an eye drop, GenTeal, which has a preservative, but the preservative is degraded rapidly in the eye and should create no allergic reaction. The advantage is in the large size bottle (15 ml) which is easier to handle and lasts longer than the individual vials.

Once the symptoms abate, you can gradually reduce the number of times you instill the drops. On a long-term basis, four times a day may turn out to be sufficient for your needs. Unless your dry eye condition is temporarily caused by a systemic disease or medication you are taking, it's very unlikely that it will ever totally disappear, so plan on a perpetual use of drops.

If your dry eye condition is beyond the help of eye drops alone, the next step would be to assess the effectiveness of a punctum plug. This is a very tiny plastic "stopper" which fits — with no discomfort — into the tear drainage opening in the inner corner of the lids. This keeps whatever moisture the tear gland produces from being rapidly drained away. It's like stoppering a sink to keep in the water even if the faucet only produces a tiny trickle. Usually, the doctor will first try a dissolvable plug to determine if that treatment will work before implanting the "permanent" plug. The procedure is very effective for most people. You won't necessarily be able to discontinue the drops, but they will remain in the eye longer and relieve much of the discomfort.

For dryness that is so severe that it's actually maiming the cornea, a soft "bandage" contact lens can be fitted to protect the cornea from erosions and pitting and the ensuing pain.

GLAUCOMA

Everybody's heard about it and some people know what it is, but no one really knows what causes the most common form — *open angle glaucoma*. To say that it is a disease character- ized by an increase in the fluid pressure within the eye would be correct, except for those few individuals whose pressure is normal, yet have glaucoma, or those whose pressure is high yet exhibit no optic nerve damage. The term "open angle" refers to the confined space or angle between the iris and cornea within the eye through which the fluid, which is continually produced, leaves the eye. (See diagram on page 10.) When that angle is open there is no physical barrier to drainage. A good way to visualize this is to think of the angle between a door and the jamb where the hinges are attached. When the door is closed there is no open space; as the door is opened, the angle gets bigger and more space is exposed. To repeat, this is all *within* the eye and has nothing to do with your tears on the outside.

Essentially, the danger of glaucoma is that it "chokes" the optic nerve, that 1/4 inch diameter bundle of about one million nerve fibers which carry vision signals from the retina to the brain. Aside from the few exceptions mentioned, a build up of pressure within the eye is the culprit. Fluid cannot be com- pressed (try compressing a water balloon) so the weakest part of the eyeball will bear the brunt of the force. This turns out to be where the optic nerve enters through the back of the eye- ball. The result is a very gradual (unnoticed by the person) loss of side vision with progressive loss to "tunnel" vision and even- tual blindness. In fact, it's the leading cause of blindness in the United States. To put this into an age perspective, the percent- ages are: under 45, about 0.1%; ages 45 to 64, about 1.5%; over 65, about 7%. Bear in mind these statistics are for diag- nosed cases and the real numbers could be much higher as you'll learn shortly. It may seem like a blessing that there is no pain associated with open angle glaucoma, but it's a blessing in disguise because pain is a warning signal of something harmful taking place.

Glaucoma tends to be hereditary in families and you need to be aware if any relatives have it and inform the doctor. Diabetics are also at higher risk. If you've ever had an eye injury be sure to tell the doctor because it can cause glaucoma — so-called secondary glaucoma — many months or years later. Some people can develop a high pressure from the long term use of steroids.

There are three very critical facts to understand about glaucoma:

1. **There is NO cure.**
2. **Any damage to the optic nerve CANNOT be reversed.**
3. **The only treatment is to lower the pressure as much as possible to prevent further vision loss.**

These facts sometimes create a dilemma for the doctor in the early stages of this disease much as a physician might have to consider in early stages of hypertension. The pressure may only be "slightly" high. Is it glaucoma? It's a well known fact that eye pressure will vary in the course of the day which means it could be normal at the time it's measured but much higher at another time, or vice versa If there is a suspicion of glaucoma, the doctor will embark on a series of specific tests. A careful analysis of the optic nerve head or photograph or digital laser image of the optic nerve head might reveal subtle destruction of nerve fibers. A detailed analysis of the peripheral field of vision test is a highly diagnostic test and indispensable. Also, the doctor will evaluate the angle using a special type of mirrored contact lens to check for any obstruction or constriction which could hinder the fluid outflow.

At what point should the doctor begin treatment? Since high pressure is the classic risk factor for glaucoma, a high pressure reading calls for initiating treatment. A loss of side vision uncovered by the peripheral field test or obvious optic nerve damage calls for treatment. On the other hand, a "slightly" high pressure with a wide-open angle and no obvious optic nerve damage, may alert the doctor to check the pressure several times throughout the day for "spikes" of high pressure. Even if it varies only a little from the "slightly" high values, some doctors will aggressively begin management before nerve damage starts. Others may decide to carefully monitor the patient for a few months before settling on a diagnosis. It is not a simple decision because the eye drops to lower the pressure have to be used every day, regularly and "forever." The cost of the medication is also a consideration.

(Because there is no pain or noticeable [at the beginning] sight loss associated with open angle glaucoma, but there are some side effects such as stinging, brow aches or difficulty seeing in low light when instilling specific eye drops, it's frequently a challenge to keep the patient adhering to the strict use schedule.)

Once the diagnosis is made, the goal is to keep the pressure as low as possible to minimize the optic nerve damage from glaucoma. There are two routes - decrease the production of fluid and/or increase the outflow. There are many medicinal eye drops available to accomplish either objective. A recently completed experimental clinical study implies that a laser procedure which places tiny holes within the iris to facilitate the outflow of fluid seems to be as effective as drops, for about the first five years, anyway. If these holes clog up, the laser may have to be used again.

Most drops will reduce the pressure 20-25%, which sounds good unless the pressure to start out with is quite high. Not all drugs work equally well on every person and as the management continues, a previously effective drug may no longer sufficiently lower the pressure to limit the nerve damage. Different or additional drugs will be prescribed. Frequent checkups are necessary to watch the pressure and monitor the field of vision loss. If vision loss continues with the maximum drug administration, surgery is necessary to create a more efficient, larger drainage route. The majority of patients do quite well with the medications, however, and never become totally blind.

What about the people who are not examined regularly, or allow years and years between thorough examinations or rely on a "screening" which simply measures the pressure at a given time of day? If these millions underwent regular, complete exams, chances are the glaucoma percentages would go up and the number of people becoming blind from glaucoma would go down.

A rare form of glaucoma is a sudden increase of pressure because of a total blockage of the outflow — *angle closure glaucoma.* You can't really miss the symptoms of a very red, painful eye, blurry vision which is often accompanied by nausea. Immediate, emergency treatment must be initiated to preserve sight.

SOMETHING IN THE EYE; CORNEAL ABRASION

These have very common symptoms: considerable pain, extreme light sensitivity, and lots of tearing. A corneal abrasion is a scraping off of part of the surface layer of the cornea which may be caused by such things as a fingernail, a tree branch, a damaged contact lens or something getting in the eye. It happens suddenly and you're very much aware of it. What you don't know, of course, is whether something is still in the eye. Get to the optometrist as soon as you can.

Because it's very difficult for the patient to keep the painful eye open, the doctor will instill an anesthetic to quiet the pain. A careful inspection will reveal if something is still stuck or embedded in the cornea which must be removed. A metallic particle can actually rust in the cornea and develop a rust ring around the particle. Surprisingly, one of the most dangerous embedded particles you can get in your eye is a piece of vegetation matter such as a grass fragment because it can open the door to a nasty fungal infection.

Once the particle is removed, you're left with an abrasion. Depending on the size and depth, this will generally heal within 36 to 72 hours. An antibiotic ointment should prevent a secondary infection in the exposed cornea. The eye may also need to be dilated and patched. The doctor will want you to return the next day to check on the healing progress and make sure there are no complications.

As soon as the anesthetic used to examine the injury wears off (about 15 minutes), pain will return. Unfortunately, the anesthetic cannot be used continually because it retards the healing process. However, there are some medications available which can dull the pain. The doctor can prescribe eyedrops and oral medications to ease your discomfort. To further ease your distress is knowing that the vast majority of these cases resolve without permanent effects on vision.

Occasionally, the healing process doesn't "anchor" the new surface cells to the underlying layers and recurrent erosions may result. Recurrent erosion means that the patch of new cells gets pulled loose much as you might pull a scab off the skin. Generally, this will happen when you wake up and open your eyes. You'll feel a sudden, sharp pain as the lid, which has become stuck to the "loose" corneal cells while you were asleep, pulls the cells loose. Overnight lubrication with ointments is needed. If this proves inadequate, hypertonic (salty) drops or ointments are prescribed to try to get better adherence of the new cells.

FLOATERS; SEEING "SPOTS"

Many people complain of noticing moving dark spots or squiggly lines in their vision. Sometimes they're described as "flies" seen out of the corner of the eyes which jump or float as you move your eyes. These objects are most noticeable when looking at a bright background such as the sky or a light colored wall.

The majority of floaters are caused by slow degenerative (aging) changes in the vitreous, the clear jelly-like material which fills the main body of the eyeball. (See illustration on page 277.) As you get older the vitreous tends to slightly shrink which produces tiny water pockets and tiny bits of solid material. These cast the shadows on the retina which are noticed as floaters. When you move your eyes, the vitreous takes a split second longer to start moving and it keeps moving a split second after your eyes stop. Think of it as a glass of water with some bits of debris in it. If you rotate the glass, the water and debris will move slower and keep moving after the glass stops. These floaters are harmless and nothing can be done to get rid of them. It's one of life's little annoyances with which you have to live.

On the other hand, a sudden appearance of floaters or a marked increase in the numbers can indicate a vitreous or retinal detachment which needs to be investigated promptly. It could lead to serious vision problems if left untreated. Another source of "dangerous" floaters could be bleeding from fragile retinal blood vessels which diabetics are very prone to develop. Finally, certain inflammatory diseases of the eye can cause deposits of white blood cells to accumulate in the vitreous and be noticed as floaters.

COMMON "RED" EYE, "PINK" EYE				
APPEARANCE	SENSATION	DISCHARGE	CAUSE	COMMENTS
			Conjunctivitis	
Moderately red lids & sclera	Burning & irritation	Watery	Viral	Recent cold, upper respiratory infection
Entire sclera somewhat red	Itching, burning	Stringy	Allergic	Puffy lids, swollen conjunctiva
Very red	Feels like something in eye	Yellowish	Bacterial	Eyelids stuck or matted
Bloody, bright red patch	Hardly any	None	Subconjunctival Hemorrhage	Sudden appearance
Very red	Considerable pain	Lots of tearing	Abrasion, Foreign Body	Very light sensitive. Can't keep eye open
Swollen lid	Tender/pain	None	Hordeolum/Stye	Upper or lower lid
Mild redness	Burning, gritty, "tired" feeling	Excessive tearing at times	Dry Eyes	Worse in wind, smoky room, low humidity
Eyelid redness	Pain, itching, burning	Crusty lid margins	Blepharitis	Frequently chronic
Lump in lid	Tightness	None	Chalazion	Can slowly enlarge

Sclera is the "white" of the eye.   *Conjunctiva* is the transparent cover overlying the sclera and inside of lids.

Glossary

Aberration:
: The failure of refracted light to focus to a common point.

Abrasion:
: An erosion of the surface cell layers. (See corneal abrasion.)

Accommodation:
: The "automatic" adjustment the eye makes in order to focus on objects at different distances.

After-image:
: An image which remains after the light stimulation to the retina has stopped. It is called positive when seen as the original, negative when dark and light are reversed or colors are seen as complimentary.

Amaurosis:
: Blindness caused by any disease.

Amblyopia:
: Poor sight in a healthy eye which does not fully improve with a corrective spectacle or contact lens. The most common type, ex-anopsia, is due to lack of use/suppression. It can also be toxic, caused by poisons.

Ametropia:
: Any sight problem caused by an improperly focused image on the retina.

Aniridia:
: A congenital lack of the iris.

Aniseikonia:
: The images seen by each eye are different in size or shape.

Anisocoria:
: The pupils are of unequal size.

Anisometropia:
: The two eyes have an unequal refractive power.

Anomalous fixation:
: An eye which uses an area other than the fovea for sighting.

Anterior chamber:
: Fluid-filled space between the cornea and the lens of the eye.

Antimetropia:
: One eye is farsighted, the other nearsighted.

Aphakia: The lens of the eye is missing.

Aqueous humor: A clear, watery fluid filling the anterior chamber. It carries nutrients to the lens and cornea, and removes waste material.

Arcus senilis: A whitish circle or arc at the border of the cornea. Very common in the aging, but harmless.

Arteriosclerosis: Hardening of the arteries.

Asthenopia: A catch-all term to describe discomfort associated with fatigue of the visual system.

Astigmatism: A refractive condition which causes parts of an object to focus at different distances behind the lens of the eye. Therefore, the entire object cannot be in focus at the same time. Usually it's caused by an "out of round" cornea.

Atrophy: The wasting away of cells or tissues from lack of nutrition.

Atropine: A drug used to temporarily dilate the pupil and paralyze accommodation.

Bifocal: A spectacle or contact lens with two focusing distances—one for far, one for near.

Binocular vision: The ability of the brain to fuse the images from each eye into a single percept.

Biomicroscope: An instrument for examining the front and interior of the eye under magnification.

Blepharitis: An inflammation of the eyelids.

Blepharospasm: A twitching of the eyelids, often due to eye strain.

Blind spot: The natural blind area of the retina where the optic nerve enters the eye.

Campimeter: An instrument for determining the integrity of the central field of vision.

Canthus: The junction of the eyelids.

Cataract:	An opaqueness in the lens of the eye.
Chalazion:	A small cyst or enlargement of a lid gland.
Choroid:	The middle-layer tissue of the eyeball.
Chromatic aberration:	A dispersion of light into its component colors.
Ciliary body:	Part of the inner layer of the eye to which the lens is attached. Contraction of the ciliary muscle permits the lens to accommodate.
Coloboma:	Congenital defect where a portion of the eye structure is missing.
Color deficiency:	The inability to correctly identify all colors.
Cone:	The light sensitive cell of the retina, mostly in the central macula region which responds to colors.
Conjunctiva:	The mucous membrane lining the "white" of the eye and the inside of the lids.
Conjunctivitis:	An inflammation of the conjunctiva.
Contrast sensitivity:	The ability of the visual system to discriminate small differences in brightness.
Convergence:	The act of rotating both eyes inward to look at a nearby object.
Contact lens:	A lens which fits directly on the front of the eye.
Cornea:	The transparent front portion of the eye.
Corneal abrasion:	An erosion of the front surface of the cornea, frequently causing pain and tearing.
Cryotherapy:	Use of intense cold to remove a cataract, seal retinal tears, destroy tumors, etc.
Crystalline lens:	The transparent, elastic lens within the eye, situated immediately behind the iris.
Cycloplegia:	A paralysis of the ciliary muscles. Suspends accommodation and dilates the pupil.

Cyclitis: An inflammation of the ciliary body.

Cylinder lens: A lens ground to give no power along one axis and maximum power at right angles to that axis.

Dacryoadenitis: An inflammation of the lacrimal gland.

Dacryocystitis: An inflammation of the lacrimal sac.

Dark focus: Change of focus of the eye in low levels of light, creating a degree of nearsightedness.

Depth perception: The quality of seeing objects as three-dimensional solids in space. True depth perception requires the brain to fuse the images from both eyes.

Diopter: The unit of measure for the power of a lens to bend light. A +1.00 lens will focus light to a point one meter away.

Diplopia: Double vision.

Divergence: Outward rotation of the eyes away from each other.

Duction: The reserve ability of the eyes to turn inward or outward and still maintain single, binocular vision.

Dyslexia: Difficulty in reading due to a brain disorder.

Ectropion: Outward eversion of the lid margin.

Edema: A tissue swelling from fluid accumulation.

Electroretinagram: Recording of the neuro-electrical responses of the entire retina to light stimulus.

Embolism: A blood vessel blocked by a clot.

Emmetropia: Light comes to a perfect focus on the retina with accommodation at rest.

Enophthalmos: A deep seated or sunken eyeball.

Entropion: Inward eversion of the lid margin.

Error of refraction: Light from a distant object does not come to a perfect focus on the retina when the eye is in a relaxed or unaccommodated state.

Esophoria: A tendency for the eyes to turn inward towards each other.

Esotropia: A crossed eye condition with one eye deviating inward.

Exophoria: A tendency for the eyes to turn outward away from each other.

Exotropia: A crossed eye condition with one eye deviating outward. Also known as "wall-eyed."

Exophthalmos: A protrusion or bulging of the eyeball.

Extrinsic muscles: The six muscles attached to the outside globe of the eye which control all eye movements.

Field of Vision: The total area of space seen by one eye (monocular) or by both eyes (binocular).

Fixation: The act of directing the visual gaze at an object in space.

Floaters: Small, solidified particles in the vitreous, which can be seen as spots or threads against any bright background.

Fluorescein: A harmless dye which glows green in ultraviolet light. Used to evaluate fit of contact lenses, condition of cornea, and retinal blood supply.

Focal point: The point at which distant light comes to a focus after being reflected or refracted.

Focal length: The distance between a lens or mirror and its focal point.

Fovea: A tiny depression in the center of the macula region of the retina. This is the area of keenest sight.

Fundus: The inside back of the eye visible with an ophthalmoscope.

Fusion:	The conversion by the brain of the images from the two eyes into one image.
Glare:	Concentrated light, much brighter than the surrounding illumination.
Glaucoma:	A disease caused by an increased fluid pressure within the eye, resulting in field of vision loss.
Gonioscopy:	A method of examining the angle between the cornea and iris in the anterior chamber.
Hemianopsia:	Blindness in one half of the visual field.
Heterochromia:	The left and right eyes each have a different color iris.
Heterophoria:	A tendency for one or both eyes to deviate or cross.
Heterotropia:	A condition wherein the eyes do not "point" together.
Hordeolum (sty):	Infection of a lash follicle of the lid margin.
Horopter:	The field of vision seen binocularly in three dimension when fixating at a given point.
Hyperemia:	Congestion of the blood vessels from an infection, inflammation, or surgery.
Hypermetropia, Hyperopia:	Farsighted. An eye whose refractive power is too weak for its length.
Hyperphoria:	A tendency for an eye to deviate upward.
Hypertensive retinopathy:	A vascular disease of the retina associated with general high blood pressure.
Hypertropia:	One eye is deviated upward.
Hypophoria:	A tendency for one eye to deviate downward.
Hypopion:	An accumulation of pus at the bottom of the anterior chamber.
Hypotropia:	One eye is deviated downward.

Infrared:	Invisible electromagnetic radiation with a wavelength just beyond visible red light. Can be felt as heat.
Intraocular tension:	The pressure of the fluid within the eye.
Iridectomy:	Surgical removal of a part of the iris.
Iris:	The thin, colored circular membrane of the eye, located in front of the lens. Its central black opening is the pupil.
Iritis:	Inflammation of the iris.
Keratitis:	Inflammation of the cornea.
Keratoconus:	Thinning of the cornea near the center, resulting in a cone-shaped bulge.
Keratometer:	An instrument for measuring the central area curvature of the cornea. Same as ophthalmometer.
Kryptok:	The name of one of the earliest types of fused bifocal lenses.
Lacrimal apparatus:	The tear-producing and disposal system of the eye.
Lagophthalmos:	An inability to fully close the lids.
Lamina cribrosa:	A perforated area of the choroid layer through which the optic nerve enters the eye.
Laser:	Acronym for Light Amplification by Stimulated Emission of Radiation, a high energy light beam capable of producing tremendous heat. By pinpointing the energy, it can be used to seal off hemorrhaging blood vessels, re-attach retinal tears, destroy eye tumors, open drainage holes for treatment of glaucoma, provide an opening in a cloudy capsule after cataract surgery, etc.
Lens:	(a) An optical device to transmit or bend light. (b) The small, transparent, circular, elastic body in the eye involved with focusing.
Lens implant:	A small plastic lens placed in the eye after removal of a cataract.

Leucoma:	A whitish opacity of the cornea.
Luxation:	A condition where the lens of the eye is displaced from its normal position.
Macropsia:	A condition where objects are seen larger than they really are.
Macula:	The most sensitive retinal area for sight and color vision.
Macular degeneration:	Partial or total loss of this sensitive retinal area (macula) resulting in reduced sight. Most common in the aged.
Micropsia:	A condition where objects are seen smaller than they really are.
Miosis:	A condition where the pupil becomes smaller.
Monocular:	Having only one eye.
Monocular vision:	Seeing with only one eye.
Muscae volitantes:	Floating spots seen against any bright background.
Multifocal:	A spectacle or contact lens with more than one focusing power area.
Mydriasis:	A condition where the pupil becomes larger.
Mydriatic:	A drug used to dilate the pupil.
Myopia:	Nearsighted. An eye whose refractive power is too strong for its length.
Near point:	The closest point which the eye is capable of accommodating. This point gradually recedes with age.
Night blindness:	An inability to see at night or in dim illumination.
Nystagmus:	Involuntary oscillation of the eye.
Oculist:	A physician who specializes in disorders and diseases of the eyes.

O.D.:

(a) Abbreviation for Latin oculus dexter, the right eye.
(b) Following a name, the degree, Doctor of Optometry.

Opacity:

Lack of transparency resulting in blockage of light. Usually refers to changes in the lens of the eye leading to cataracts.

Ophthalmologist:

A medical specialist dealing primarily with diseases and surgery of the eyes.

Ophthalmometer:

An instrument for measuring the central area curvature of the cornea. Same as keratometer.

Ophthalmoplegia:

Widespread paralysis of the eye muscles.

Ophthalmoscope:

An instrument used to inspect the inside of the eye.

Optic atrophy:

Degeneration of the optic nerve fibers with partial or complete sight loss.

Optic disc:

The area of the retina where the optic nerve and blood supply enters the eye.

Optic nerve:

The collection of about one million nerve fibers connecting each eye to the brain.

Optician:

A person who grinds lenses and/or dispenses optical goods.

Optometrist:

A specialist skilled in the detection of eye diseases; in the diagnosis and treatment of disorders of the eyes and visual system.

Orbit:

The bony socket which surrounds the eye.

Orthophoria:

Straight eyes without any tendency for either eye to deviate.

Orthoptics:

Scientifically planned eye exercises to straighten the eyes and develop binocularity.

O.S.:

Abbreviation for Latin oculus sinister, left eye.

O.U.:

Abbreviation for Latin oculus uterque, both eyes.

Papillitis:	An inflammation of the optic disc.
Paresis:	A slight or partial paralysis.
Perimetry:	The measurement of the extent and integrity of the visual field.
Peripheral vision:	The ability to perceive objects and movements away from the direct line of sight.
Photophobia:	An intolerance to light.
Photopsia:	Seeing flashing lights which are not physically present.
Pinguecula:	A small, yellowish elevation on the conjunctiva.
Pink eye:	A common term for an acute conjunctivitis.
Pleoptics:	Light stimulation therapy in the treatment of amblyopia.
Presbyopia:	Decreased ability of the eye, with age, to focus near objects and printed material.
Prism:	A lens which displaces or bends light in one direction.
Pterygium:	A triangular shaped, vascular growth on the conjunctiva near the limbus, which may overgrow the cornea.
Ptosis:	A drooping of the upper lid.
Pupil:	The small, black circular opening in the iris through which light enters the eye.
Refraction:	The bending of light as it passes from a medium of one density to that of another.
Refractive error:	A defect in the refractive system of the eye which prevents light from coming to a clear, sharp focus on the retina.
Retina:	The inner layer of the eye containing the light sensitive cells and numerous nerve cells.

Retinopathy:	Changes in the retina as a result of disease or inflammation.
Retinoscope:	An instrument used to measure the refractive power of the eye objectively.
Retrobulbar neuritis:	An inflammation of the optic nerve behind the optic disc.
Rods:	The light sensitive cells of the retina which respond to light, dark, movements, shapes, but not to colors.
Saccade:	A quick, ballistic movement of the eye from one point to another.
Sclera:	The outer white covering of the eye.
Scotoma:	A blind or partially missing area in the visual field.
Snellen chart:	A letter or number chart for scientifically measuring the central visual acuity.
Slit lamp:	See biomicroscope.
Squint:	(a) To look with the eyes partially closed. (b) A deviating eye.
Stereopsis:	Seeing objects in three dimension. The end result of the brain fusing the images from both eyes.
Strabismus:	The two eyes are not "pointing" together. Concomitant, when the eyes move together even though one is deviated; non-concomitant (paralytic), when the deviating eye does not move together with the pointing eye.
Sty:	The common name for hordeolum.
Subluxation:	Partially displaced lens of the eye.
Synechia:	Adhesion of the iris to the lens or cornea.
Tachistoscope:	An instrument used in visual therapy to enlarge the span of visual recognition.
Tangent screen:	An instrument used to examine the central visual field for scotomas and other abnormalities.

Tear film:	Thin fluid layer which covers the cornea and eye.
Temple:	The arm or handle of an eyeglass frame which fits over the ear.
Thrombosis:	Blood clot obstruction in a vessel.
Tonometer:	An instrument for measuring the fluid pressure within the eye.
Trachoma:	A viral disease of the conjunctival lining of the lids resulting in a cobblestone appearance and causing scarring of the cornea.
Trichiasis:	A condition in which the eyelashes grow inward towards the cornea.
Trifocal:	A lens with three distinct focusing areas.
Tropia:	A deviated or crossed eye.
Uvea:	The choroid, ciliary body and iris of the eye.
Uveitis:	An inflammation of the uvea.
Ultraviolet:	Highly energetic, invisible electromagnetic radiation with a wavelength adjacent to visible violet. Responsible for skin tanning; can cause eye damage.
Visual acuity:	The sharpness of sight, usually measured in the Snellen fractions 20/20, 20/80, etc.
Visual axis:	Direction of gaze.
Visual evoked response:	Minute electrical current generated by the visual cortex in response to light stimulation of the macular region of the retina.
Visual illusion:	Misinterpretation by the brain of a visual setting or scene.
Vitrectomy:	The removal of cloudy vitreous humor and its replacement with a clear fluid.
Vitreous humor:	A transparent, jelly-like substance which fills the eye behind the lens.

Vertical phoria: The tendency for an eye to deviate upward or downward.

Visual Therapy: Various types of scientific training procedures geared to improve the functioning of the visual system.

Wall eyed: One eye deviates outward.

Xanthelasma: A flat yellowish growth on the lids.

Xerosis: Abnormal dryness of the eye.

Zonule of Zinn: Thin, threadlike ligaments which hold the lens in place within the eye.

Index

A

Abrasion, Corneal 119, 273
Accommodation 39, 40, 42
Acuity, Visual 37, 71, 141
Aging, Vision 45, 46, 78-9
AIDS 144
Albinism 24
Allergies 122, 260
Amblyopia 27, 71, 145, 174
Amsler Grid 69-70
Aqueous Humor 11
Arcus Senilis 272
Arteriosclerosis 277
Astigmatism 44, 78-9

B

Bifocal 79, 85-87
Binocular Vision 63, 162
Bioptic Telescope 251
Blepharitis 270
Blind Spot 14
Blindness, Legal 235-6, 247
Blindness, Temporary 267, 293
Bulging Eyes 67, 279
Burns 266-7

C

Cataract 143, 220, 276
Chalazion 270
Children's Vision 63
Choroid 10
Choroiditis 278
Ciliary Muscle 11
Coloboma 275
Color Vision 31-3, 71
Cones 13
Conjunctiva 272
Conjunctivitis 272, 283

Contrast Sensitivity 69
Convergence 41, 142, 151
Cornea 10, 73, 107
Corneal Ulcer 274
Corneal Sensitivity 67, 127
Crossed Eyes 47, 63, 145, 172

D

Dacryocystitis 271
Depth Perception 17, 19, 148
Developmental Vision 163
Diabetes 223
Diabetic Retinopathy 215, 223, 277
Dilation 62-3
Diopter 78
Directionality 164
Dislocated Lens 276
Distorted Vision 70
Double Vision 67, 151-2, 224
Drops 62-3
Dry Eyes 64-6, 130, 220
Dyslexia 159

E

Ectropion 271
Electro-diagnostic Tests 71-4
Electroretinogram 71
Enophthalmos 279
Entropion 271
Episcleritis 274
Examination, visual 58-63
Exophthalmos 279
Eye Glasses 77-9, 80-4
Eye Movements 37-41
Eye Muscles 14-5
Eye Pain 119, 124
Eye Pressure, see Glaucoma
Eyeball 10, 17

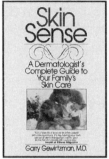
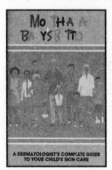
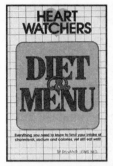
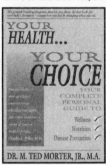